"This historical account of one state's journey to introduce an expanded role for qualified nurses is exceptionally well written, interesting in its detail, well documented, and historically valuable—not only as a historical piece, but also as a great teaching tool. It lends itself to analyzing, synthesizing, and applying a theoretical framework of change and other theoretical constructs. This story of change describes in detail the strategies, logistics and tactics (personal, professional, political, and social) of a change process that was successful."

Loretta C. Ford, EdD, PNP
Cofounder of the 1ˢᵗ NP
Program in the country

"Freund vividly brings to life her own and others' lived experience through captivating first-person accounts of why and how North Carolina's first nurse practitioners were ushered into being. Her rich narrative, contextual insights, and retrospective analyses are both revelatory and instructive to contemporary nurse practitioners. The levers of change deftly used by Freund and her co-creators—collegial relationships among and between nurses and physicians; professional organizational policy development; and strategic connections to political power—are just as relevant and basic today. Freund's retrospective is a reminder that North Carolina nurse practitioners have yet to fulfill the potential of our extraordinary origin story. It is simultaneously a tribute to our remarkable past and a thunderous call to action for full practice authority."

Gale Adcock, FNP,
N.C. House Representative

A NEW
ORDER
OF
THINGS

Sara —
From what I know of you, I believe
you are a kind and honorable woman.
I think you'll enjoy reading about some
of the social activists described herein.
Enjoy, Cindy

A NEW ORDER OF THINGS

The Origins of a Nurse
Practitioner Movement

Cindy

Cynthia Freund

Library of Congress Cataloging-in-Publication Data
Names: Freund, Cynthia M., author. | University of North Carolina at Chapel Hill. School of Nursing, issuing body.
Title: A new order of things : origins of a nurse practitioner movement / Cynthia Freund.
Description: [Chapel Hill, North Carolina] : The University of North Carolina at Chapel Hill School of Nursing, [2022] | Includes bibliographical references.
Identifiers: LCCN 2022022510 | ISBN 9781469672861 (paperback) | ISBN 9781469672878 (ebook)
Subjects: LCSH: University of North Carolina at Chapel Hill. School of Nursing--History. | Nurse practitioners--North Carolina--History. | Nurse practitioners--Training of--North Carolina--History.
Classification: LCC RT82.8 .F74 2022 | DDC 610.7306/92071175659--dc23/eng/20220608
LC record available at https://lccn.loc.gov/2022022510

C. Glenn Pickard, MD—*The Founder of North Carolina's Nurse Practitioner Movement*

Many helped move the nurse practitioner concept from an innovation to a thriving advanced practice role, now a mainstay of the health care system. One person, though, C. Glenn Pickard, stands out as the most passionate and dedicated champion of nurse practitioners, and is considered by most the founder of North Carolina's nurse practitioner movement.

Lucy Conant, RN, PhD—*A Founding Partner in North Carolina's Nurse Practitioner Movement*

Nurse practitioner programs of the late 1960s and 1970s were founded by nurse–physician teams. Neither alone could have established a viable program. Lucy Conant came to the University of North Carolina School of Nursing as a new dean with the intention of developing a nurse practitioner program. Such commitment from the nursing school dean was an ingredient essential to the success of North Carolina's nurse practitioner movement.

Audrey Joyce Booth, RN, MSN—*A Stalwart Advocate*

Audrey Booth was a mentor to many nurses in North Carolina for over twenty years. She guided and advised those who became leaders in the nurse practitioner movement, as well as those who became leaders in other areas of nursing and health care. She faithfully guarded nurse practitioners' legal status and fought to maintain a delicate alliance between the long-standing nursing and medical regulatory boards of the state.

UNC's First Nurse Practitioner Graduates—*The Pioneers*

They risked becoming nurse practitioners because they believed it was right and would be good for nursing. Despite at times doubting the wisdom of their decision, in the end they were proud nurse practitioner graduates of the first class—the pilot class of 1970. They stood at the forefront of the movement in North Carolina.

There is nothing more difficult to take in hand, more perilous to conduct, or more uncertain in its success, than to take the lead in the introduction of a new order of things. He who innovates has for enemies all those who have done well under the existing order of things, and only lukewarm supporters in those who may do well under the new....

From *The Prince,*
Niccolò Machiavelli
(1469–1527)

TABLE OF CONTENTS

ACKNOWLEDGMENTS

I am grateful to many, but I offer my utmost gratitude to Glenn Pickard and Audrey Booth, the two people who got me started on my professional journey. Glenn first whetted my appetite to become a nurse practitioner. We quickly bonded as colleagues because we both loved the political side of moving this nurse practitioner innovation into the mainstream of North Carolina's health care system. We were both activists at heart, and he was a loyal supporter throughout our endeavors. Audrey Booth was a mentor in the most genuine sense. She showed me how all things "political" worked and helped me mature professionally in many ways. She soon became a lifelong friend, and for forty-seven years Audrey helped me be a stronger person professionally and personally. She lived one month shy of ninety-three years and was a life role model for almost five decades. I regret neither lived long enough to see this book in published form. Glenn and Audrey both awakened me to my adult purpose.

The friends I developed at Penn have remained my friends. Joan Lynaugh, Barbara Bates, Karen Wilkerson, and Neville Strump all valued history. Our discussions of nursing and medical history, especially around a dinner table complemented by wine, engendered many lively debates. And in that loving and congenial company, my desire to write North Carolina's nurse practitioner story was renewed. I am grateful for that intellectual prod I always experienced when with them, and just as strongly, I value the fun, friendship, and love we have shared and continue to share.

Many others also helped me bring the book to press. My former administrative assistant, Karen Hearne, came to my rescue once again, transcribing tapes, editing transcripts, and making order out of the stacks of papers I had collected related to this project. Betty Hughes, a dear friend, completed most of the first and second rounds of transcript editing. David Hughes, one night while talking about the book, recited an apt quotation from *The Prince*—which I could remember only in concept, but which he recalled word for word, and ultimately is used as the epigraph for this book.

Several people offered, or graciously agreed, to read an early version of the book in its entirety—Jane Arndt, Betty Compton, Linda Cronenwett, Patricia D'Antonio, Ruth Efird, Celia Sandford, Margarete Sandelowski, Joanna Selim, Margaret Wilkman, and SeonAe Yeo. Linda Cronenwett has been a colleague, and mostly a friend, since the '80s. I have always loved her writing and especially how she puts thoughts together with such insight and clarity. Over the years, we've had many spirited but friendly debates about nursing and the health care system. Margarete Sandelowski came to UNC in 1986. I have always valued her critical thinking. Patricia D'Antonio gave freely of her time to read an early draft and provided advice about the world of publishing. Linda, Margarete, and Patricia provided especially thoughtful critiques.

Agnes Binder-Weisinger, a graduate of the third class of family nurse practitioners at UNC, caught wind of this project just as I was realizing how expensive this endeavor was becoming. Her financial gift to the School of Nursing Foundation for the Nurse Practitioner History Project helped defray the costs of converting cassette tapes to MP3 digital format and hiring transcriptionists to convert audio format to the written word. Her generosity has been a great boost.

Linda Whitney Hobson served as my editor and provided substantive editing, and importantly, positive encouragement. Because we were working together during the pandemic, we did not meet in person—but we did get to know each other more personally through phone and email conversations—a definite value-added gift. Although I am not grateful for the pandemic of 2020, it did allow me to hide out at home and write.

Most importantly, I am extraordinarily fortunate and grateful for my wife and life partner, Ruth Ouimette. I spent most of every day with my head in papers or my fingers pecking away on the computer, while Ruth took on many of my responsibilities, which gave me more time to focus on research and writing. Even more significantly, she read the first draft of every chapter and section of the book, and every other version after the first. She, as an early nurse practitioner, knew the content. She completed the Bates and Lynaugh Adult Nurse Practitioner Program at the University of Rochester in 1972 and joined the UNC faculty in 1975. She was the only one willing to say "good," "good, but see my comments," or "not so great, start over." She is a gutsy lady, but only in the kindest of ways.

Ruth understood my commitment to finish this book, and she wanted to support me to do so in whatever way she could—as she has always done. We met in 1975 when she joined the nurse practitioner faculty at UNC. Ruth played a role in the North Carolina nurse practitioner story, too, but she also has the lead role in my own life story.

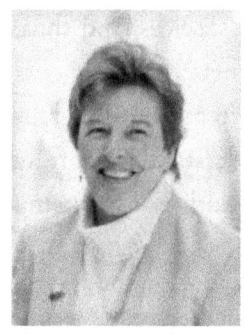

E ager for something new and challenging, seven years after graduating from nursing school I decided to return to school for a graduate degree in nursing. I didn't know exactly "what" the new and challenging would be, but I knew I would know it when I saw it. Fortunately, I chose the School of Nursing at the University of North Carolina at Chapel Hill (UNC), where I enrolled as a graduate student in the fall of 1970. From that point on through 1984, I became involved in leading and establishing the North Carolina nurse practitioner movement. That, the nurse practitioner movement, was the new and challenging.

After my first three months of searching for a path, my faculty advisor Faye Pickard sent me to her husband, Dr. Glenn Pickard—the founder and medical codirector of the UNC Family Nurse Practitioner (FNP) Program. When we first met, he and I talked for two hours—rather, he talked, and I listened with rapt attention. A colorful storyteller, he described the past five years of political maneuvering it had taken to get the program approved, funded, and off the ground. Glenn's zeal was contagious, and I caught it.

My graduate clinical courses involved informal nurse practitioner (NP) training with Glenn and Dr. James (Jim) Bryan in the hospital clinics. However, my petition to enroll in the FNP Program for graduate course credit failed because the faculty would not approve graduate credit for those "doctor-taught" courses. I finished my course work, and returned home in 1972 to Milwaukee, Wisconsin, to write my thesis—a study of the first nurse practitioners in a rural clinic in North Carolina. Seven months later, I returned to UNC to defend my thesis, and that summer, in July 1973, I was back in North Carolina to set up a pilot satellite FNP program. For my rich and intense early exposure to the concept of "nurse practitioners," I thank Faye Pickard, Glenn Pickard, and Jim Bryan for lighting a flame in my thinking.

After the pilot, and for the next five years, I served as associate director of the FNP Program, as well as the area health education center liaison for NP programs, and coordinator of the North Carolina Consortium of NP Programs. By 1978, opposition and barriers to the utilization of nurse practitioners were raised by skeptics in the guise of economic issues. More nurse practitioners would deliver more services, and thus, the overall cost of health care and insurance would increase, opponents said. Many of these economic arguments felt hollow to me, but I had no counterargument. I felt that some of us needed to understand more fully and be able to speak the language of economics and health care financing to counter those arguments.

Therefore, in 1978, I left Chapel Hill and enrolled in a new PhD program, one with a combined focus on health and business administration. It was a perfect match for what I needed and wanted—a focused study of finance and economics. For my dissertation research, I compared productivity and cost per patient between a physician-only practice and three different nurse practitioner practice settings, all in North Carolina. My cumulative experiences with the UNC FNP Program to date had been career changing and life altering.

After completing my PhD requirements, I went to the University of Pennsylvania (also referred to as simply "Penn") to start a new program, a joint degree program leading to a PhD in Nursing and an MBA from The Wharton School. This project presented a new challenge, one I rather relished. The first hurdle in getting this program off the ground was to convince the mostly male Wharton faculty that, indeed, nurses would be able to successfully complete the Wharton courses—just as other MBA students did. Furthermore, the innovativeness of this first-of-its-kind program was alluring to the change agent in me.

A year or so earlier, before coming to Penn, I competed for and was awarded funding from the Leonard Davis Institute of Health Economics, The Wharton School, for my doctoral dissertation. This connection subsequently facilitated my interactions with the health system faculty at Wharton and with leading health economists. In some ways, it was comparable to a post-doc fellowship, making my time at Penn a time of professional maturation.

While at Penn, I maintained close contact with Audrey Booth, a mentor to me during my time with the Family Nurse Practitioner Program at UNC. We often talked about what made the North Carolina nurse practitioner effort successful yet different from some of the other early programs. We decided to record conversations with the founders, pioneers, and advocates of North Carolina's Nurse Practitioner Program—thirty-three of them in total—over three years. Audrey had indeed planted the seed for this book. However, she was not interested in writing the book, so I soon took up the project on my own.

In 1984 I returned to UNC as department chair, and then, five years later I became dean of the School of Nursing. I retired in 2001; actually, I often say I retired then from paid employment. I had moved three times, each time taking the interview cassette tapes and collection of research material with me, and each time vowing, "I need to write this book!" Finally, by 2014, I began to do so. At first, I phased the project. From 2014 to 2016, the cassette tape recordings were digitized, then transcribed, and then properly edited. In mid-2017, I started the final transcript editing process, verifying names, entering clarifying notes, and making notes and timelines for myself, as the pertinent "conversations" would become prime source material for this book. It dawned on me one day that the fiftieth anniversary of the UNC Nurse Practitioner Program would be in 2020—only eighteen months or so into the future. And suddenly it registered that of the many involved with the movement, only two of us who could write this book were still living. With that shock, I worked nonstop until the book manuscript was completed in 2022.

I spent all but the first seven years of my professional life associated with renowned institutions of higher learning. That makes me an academic, perhaps not your typical academic but an academic, nonetheless. What I loved most was teaching, leading, mentoring, and challenging people to think differently, to question what is, and to imagine what could be.

Therefore, don't expect this book to be a typical "historical tome." Do expect it to be about the time, place, and people *who did* think differently, questioned what was, and imagined what else could be. Do expect it to be written in narrative style, making it enticing to read. And do expect it to be about the careful and continuous tending of both proponents and opponents of change and innovation required to introduce "a new order of things," the nurse practitioner movement's origins in the early 1970s.

CHAPTER ONE

Introduction

A NEW ORDER OF THINGS:
POLITICS AND RELATIONSHIPS

"All politics is local" is a well-known adage of Thomas P. "Tip" O'Neill, Jr., a long-serving and well-respected former member of the U.S. House of Representatives. When advising nurses about political advocacy, North Carolina Representative Gale Adcock, RN, FNP, added in 2021, "All politics is relationship-driven."[1] Both comments are apt dictums befitting the North Carolina nurse practitioner movement: it was political, it was local, and it was relationship driven.

No matter the scale of change, it is a political process driven by relationship building and relationship nurturing. There are no four steps to making change. There are no easy steps. Change is a nuanced process. Innovators and change agents must be strategists, with both short-term strategies and long-term end goals. They must be adept at recognizing subtle clues and nimble enough to take advantage of an opportune moment or event. They think ahead and of the present moment simultaneously. Their change, their innovation is their passion.

A New Order of Things provides many lessons on change and innovation adoption, lessons told through the stories of the core innovators who took the nurse practitioner idea from a clinic experiment to a university program at the University of North Carolina at Chapel Hill and extended that to two additional educational programs across the state of North Carolina, and to a partnership with community leaders developing rural clinics dotting its rural state. The NP movement in North Carolina involved more than a change in nursing practice. It also involved a change in how medical and nursing professional associations and regulatory bodies interacted. It required a partnership with rural communities seeking primary care services. It required a change in how nurses and physicians worked together.

A New Order of Things: The Origins of a Nurse Practitioner Movement is a story of change and innovation at the organizational, health system, and state level from the mid-sixties to the mid-seventies. The story is told in the form of traditional narrative history[2]—through the voices of the leaders of North Carolina's nurse practitioner movement. And, as importantly, it has contemporary relevance. It is a book of interest to nurse practitioner students, to health practitioners wanting to make change in their practice organizations and the health system, and to nursing and medical historians as well.

THE NORTH CAROLINA NURSE PRACTITIONER MOVEMENT

At its beginnings, the nurse practitioner movement was not a national movement. In fact, it started, despite opposition from the national organizations representing nursing and medicine, because it bore the strength and cohesion of a local movement at its inception. From the mid-sixties to the early seventies, many nurse practitioner-like experiments began within states, in a variety of local communities—some being almost as local as one can get. These experiments dotted the country, from the western states of California and Washington to Denver, Colorado, and New Mexico, to the middle of the country in Memphis, Tennessee, and Kentucky, and into the eastern states of North Carolina, New York, Massachusetts, and Maine—to name just a few.

North Carolina's "New Order of Things" started as an experiment in a clinic of the University of North Carolina (UNC) Medical Center in 1965. Nursing and medical leaders were finding new and more valuable ways to build on the extant clinical knowledge and skills of nurses in order to provide more effective comprehensive continuing care. Even though at that time there was no reference to the title "nurse practitioner," these continuing care clinic experiments were the genesis of the Nurse Practitioner Program at UNC. When local community leaders came to the university seeking help to bring health care services to their communities where there were none, the continuing care clinic experiment morphed into the Family Nurse Practitioner Program.

The University of North Carolina at Chapel Hill Family Nurse Practitioner (FNP) Program was one of the early FNP programs, admitting its pilot class in September 1970. Students from the pilot class were destined for practice in three clinics serving rural counties surrounding Chapel Hill. In the next two years, students were admitted to the program from the western, central, and eastern parts of North Carolina. By 1974, North Carolina's nurse practitioner movement was firmly ensconced in multiple local communities across the state.

The new nurse practitioner role not only changed the way nurses and physicians related to each other; it also pushed the boundaries of nursing into territory claimed and fiercely protected by physicians. This realignment of nursing and medical responsibilities was a threat to many, and as a result, not all nurses and physicians supported this new breed of nurses. Some were adamantly opposed. Therefore, the state regulatory boards of both professions and the state and local professional societies had to be informed; their affiliative support, as well as legislative support, was important to the success of nurse practitioners.

Over the past one hundred years, realignment of the practice boundaries between physicians and nurses has been considerable and almost continuous. One time long ago, the blood pressure cuff and stethoscope were the sole prerogative of the physician. Today, almost anyone can lay claim to the prerogative of blood pressure measurement—including patients themselves. This example oversimplifies how nurses and physicians have negotiated their boundaries of responsibility and authority, but it does show how "ownership" of specific knowledge and skills migrates over time.

Determinations of power, responsibility, and authority are shaped by social, political, and economic forces, some of them beyond the control of either nurses or physicians. Certainly the "tools of the trade"—the stethoscope, otoscope, ultrasound, or other evolving technologies—are not the main determinants of boundary specification. They may be the most visible, especially to the public, but they do not represent the crux of boundary changes among nurses and physicians that accompanied the nurse practitioner movement. Task delegation is not a crucial element of boundary specification either. Physicians understand task delegation; they have used it often, especially when they want to free themselves from certain tasks. Yankauer and Sullivan point out that physical examinations had not been previously so delegated, but this, too, could be accepted by physicians without fear of proprietary encroachment by nurse practitioners. They argue, however, that "sharing the primal role of diagnostician and therapist, even though theoretically under the aegis of a physician and with physician consultation and backup readily available, was more difficult to accept."[3]

Fortunately, other leading physicians saw boundary "sharing" differently. Julie Fairman, in her analysis of the nurse practitioner movement nationally, describes its development during the '60s and '70s

as a growing informal coalition of nurses and physicians who saw the idea of working together as a fundamental way to improve patient care. [The movement] altered professional boundaries...and reshaped clinical practice, particularly outside of hospitals, and provided the foundation for questioning who had the authority to provide care to particular patients at particular times and places.[4]

To create a new and better order of things, one must disrupt the old order—and for that, one will surely make enemies and face vocal opposition just as much today as it was in Machiavellian times. But one can also make and nurture new friends and allies who will join in the new order. And that is precisely what the early proponents of the North Carolina nurse practitioner movement did. They built relationships with nurses, physicians, legislators, lawyers, influential leaders in the health professions, and local community leaders. Not only did they develop these relationships, but they also nourished them, thereby making new allies. The result was a spiraling coalition of supporters who took the North Carolina nurse practitioner movement statewide.

The boundary expansion by nurse practitioners changed nursing practice dramatically and forever. Nurse practitioners ushered in advanced practice clinical roles. They changed the dynamic between nurses and patients by having direct access to patients and by the decision-making authority to diagnose and prescribe, all complementing the positive and holistic relationship nurses had always had with patients. Furthermore, nurse practitioners and their physician colleagues changed the doctor–nurse relationship to one based on common goals and respect for the knowledge of the other. Taken together, over time, these changes in both nursing and medical practice constituted a movement—a concentrated effort by a few to change how primary care was provided in this country and how nurses and physicians would and could work together. The nurse practitioner movement ushered in the concept of advanced nursing practice.

That and more is the subject of this book. In North Carolina, the nurse practitioner movement was indeed local, many times over, and by necessity and proclivity it was relationship driven.

A NARRATIVE OF MANY: *THE CONVERSATIONS COLLECTION*[5]

I was involved with the Family Nurse Practitioner Program at UNC in various positions from 1970 to 1981, first as a graduate student, then as associate director of the program, and as coordinator of the Consortium for Statewide NP Programs. I conducted the first study of NPs in North Carolina, and a few years later for my dissertation research, I evaluated the economic impact of NPs in different types of practice settings. To many of us involved with bringing the nurse practitioner innovation into the mainstream of health care services in North Carolina, our work was our passion. Day or night, we would do whatever it took to advance acceptance of nurse practitioners and defend them from adversarial opponents.

Many people made substantial contributions to the nurse practitioner movement in North Carolina, and the account of their involvement brings life and detail to the story. Between 1982 and 1984, approximately ten years after the movement's beginning, Audrey Booth, a mentor, colleague, and friend, and I held "conversations" with thirty-plus key individuals involved in North Carolina's nurse practitioner movement. We call these discussions "conversations"—instead of interviews—because it would have been difficult and cumbersome to conduct formal interviews with those whom we had worked with so intensely during the formative years of the nurse practitioner movement in North Carolina. Yet these conversations serve as primary source material throughout the book, and as such, the book is a narrative told by many.

This book, then, can be described as narrative history—the writing of history in story-based form. That does not mean the book is without analysis and evidence. All these elements—narrative, analysis, and evidence—are woven together. Sometimes, the narrative will read like a story and, in fact, may be a story. This is inevitable because storytelling is embedded in the fabric of southern culture—and many of the interviewees and those involved in the nurse practitioner movement were southerners as well as great storytellers. As one of the non-southerners involved, I did learn to appreciate how a story can leave the reader with the context, emotion, and dynamics of an experience, as well as how it can also provide an analysis and interpretation of events. The narratives of the founders and champions of the North Carolina nurse practitioner movement allowed me to describe and show the emotionally revealing and more fascinating aspects of the politically nuanced and highly charged process of bringing the nurse practitioner innovation to widespread adoption in the state of North Carolina.

In the first part of the book, and throughout most of the book, I use the third-person point of view to describe context and events; in these instances, I was not the significant actor or informant; I am providing background, context, and interpretation. However, there are times when I am the key or sole informant, and therefore have no choice but to switch to first-person point of view. I provide this advance warning here as such a change in voice can be unsettling to readers.

A PARADIGM FOR CHANGE AND INNOVATION

This book is not only a history of North Carolina's nurse practitioner movement. It is a lesson on how to counter the dangers of and resistance to any innovation. The story of how the nurse practitioner movement was so quickly accepted and spread throughout North Carolina offers a paradigm on how to advocate and garner support for an innovation that has systemwide effects, as most innovations will have such effects no matter how large or small the system. Further, most innovations will have supporters and adversaries, and both must be attended early in the process of implementing change if an innovation is to succeed.

Extensive preplanning is also requisite. So too is a sensitivity to recognize unexpected opportunities, followed by the courage to act on one's instinct and belief that an unexpected opportunity is just "what the doctor ordered"—or "what the nurse practitioner ordered." There is no roadmap; there is only the constant realization of the end goal and the commitment to make as many needed twists and turns in order to get there. We often referred to this as "political instinct" and "a nose that knows," and we often adjusted our plans in order to follow those noses.

The book starts with a brief look into the first day of the first class of the Family Nurse Practitioner Program at the University of North Carolina at Chapel Hill in September 1970, showing how the seven students were found and recruited to this pilot class. And we will be introduced to the two lead founders of the nurse practitioner movement in North Carolina.

After that snapshot, we will go back to the mid-1960s to review the societal context of the times, the national health care system, and the need for expanded health care services. From there, we will move to the local context, first at the environment within the University Health Affairs Division that provided fertile ground for innovative and nontraditional approaches to solving societal health problems. Second, we will examine the state of health services in local communities to see how they organized themselves to find their own solutions to inadequate health care services.

All the above sets the stage for the evolving development of a nurse practitioner program at UNC, to the development of statewide programs for nurse practitioners, and ultimately to a statewide nurse practitioner movement. Nudging a program that teaches nurses to become nurse practitioners into a statewide movement that changes health care delivery as well as the relationship among nurses, physicians, and other health care professionals, involves more than the educational program alone. Professional associations and legal authorities also had a stake in these changes, and their natural tendency was to respond to protect their vested interests and preserve their boundaries—Machiavelli's existing "order of things."

At this point, the story culminates with a description and examination of an ever-expanding network of advocates and proponents that brought all the forces together in concert to orchestrate the Nurse Practitioner Program into a nurse practitioner movement. The concert was not always in perfect harmony, but it played on to finish its movement. The book ends in an epilogue where all the early 1970 innovations are brought up to date, not omitting a look at two nagging conundrums: degree muddle and boundary shifting.

The lessons on how to effect change, how to create a new order of things, are provided through narrating the origins of the nurse practitioner movement in North Carolina, the ideas, and actions of the people—the founders, movers, and shakers of the NP movement in North Carolina, and their aspirations, motivations, vested interests, and myriad roles. The story tells of organizations, their commitments, and their competitive and cooperative relationships. It is also about the growing professionalism of medicine and nursing, at its best and its worst.

It is a story of politics—power plays, negotiation, compromise, hidden agendas, and backroom decisions. It is also the story of the network of people and organizations trying to improve health care in North Carolina. Altogether, these historical events, facts, and human decisions and actions tell the story of the nurse practitioner movement in North Carolina. And through North Carolina's story, the book provides a blueprint and tactics on how to make change and move an innovation to widespread adoption.

CHAPTER TWO

The First Day

On the morning of September 8, 1970, a group of seven nurses found their way across the sprawling, historic, green campus of the University of North Carolina at Chapel Hill to a fifth-floor classroom in Carrington Hall, a recently dedicated building for the School of Nursing. The fall semester of 1970 was the first time Carrington Hall was open for students and classes. September 8 was also noteworthy, for it was the "First Day" of the first family nurse practitioner program in North Carolina.

Most of these seven were either strangers or distant acquaintances to one another. Even so, they were about to spend five days a week over the next five months together—and they would get to know each other quite well. At this point, however, all they knew about each other was that they were nurses embarking on an exciting yet risky professional endeavor.

For these seven, it was risky for several reasons. Most of their peers were dead set against this so-called family nurse practitioner (FNP) idea. Nurses across the country thought those who supported this newly expanded nursing role were selling out to physicians. Opponents also believed that nurses had finally begun to realize some independence from doctors, but to them, the FNP role threatened these newfound gains. Further, the doubters presumed that nurse practitioners would become mini-doctors, forgoing their nursing identity and values. Nursing faculty were particularly opposed to this new role, but some nurses in clinical practice also held similar views. One of them described her first and very personal experience with such opposition.

> The dean of my nursing school would not write a reference because she was worried and didn't support [the NP role]...expressing that very clearly in our conversations. I decided I had to accept that. It was worth the challenge, and if there was anything that I needed to prove, it was to myself. I wouldn't necessarily have to change what I was taught and what I believed in; I would just do a better job and stretch my arms a little farther and use my head a little more.[1]

Others in the classroom had experienced similar snubs from their peers, teachers, and superiors in the field.

It was not just the majority of nurses who were opposed to nurse practitioners. Physicians were as well, some fearing competition, others a loss of supervisory control. And the professional associations of both medicine and nursing were vocal in their opposition—except in North Carolina, where the North Carolina Nurses Association was supportive. Considering all this opposition, why did these initial seven even show up on September 8, 1970?

Because they were risk takers and pioneers. They wanted changes in the scope of their practice. They knew they could do more. In fact, they often did more, even though taking on more responsibility was not sanctioned or legitimized. They were tired of playing the "doctor–nurse game."[2] They knew the health care system had to change. And in various ways, they all had gradually moved toward taking on expanded responsibilities in their daily practice and even in their daily lives.

Compton, one of the seven who lived in a rural community without a local physician, described how she would often come home from work, after the usual clinic or doctor's office hours, of course, to find a mother with a sick child sitting on her porch. The mother was there for advice: should she take the child to the emergency room, call a doctor for a prescription, or do such and such at home? Compton encountered similar situations almost daily as a practicing public health nurse. Most of the other nurses there in that classroom had experienced similar situations.

As they came into the classroom, the first seven introduced themselves to each other: Evelyn Aabel, June Baise, Betty Compton, Ruth Efird, Sandra Hogan, Phoebe Hood, and Margaret Wilkman. Introductions and conversations were a bit stiff and tense—but that would never be so again. Then Dr. Glenn Pickard, medical codirector of the FNP Program, and Dr. Lucy Conant, dean of the School of Nursing at the University of North Carolina at Chapel Hill, came and greeted them.

This welcome was, to these nurses, a formidable one. Even though they had some idea of their undertaking, it was a rather amorphous understanding. They knew or at least thought or hoped this new role would be great for nursing as well as for all those patients they knew who needed a better system of care. They also knew they were risking their professional careers and reputations, and their means of livelihood, by being the first to step forward—and yet here they were. Pickard and Conant were apprehensive on this day as well, but for different reasons—it was called a "pilot" program intentionally. Yet they did not share their apprehension with the students; what they did share were their enthusiasm and excitement.

Glenn Pickard had been working on the nurse practitioner idea since 1965 when he returned to UNC following his internship in New York and a tour of naval service. Pickard is considered the "founder of the North Carolina nurse practitioner movement" to all those associated with and graduating from the Nurse Practitioner Program during the '70s. He had been working with nurses in the North Carolina Memorial Hospital clinics for the past five years, helping them advance their knowledge, skills, and responsibilities in clinical care.[3] He also advocated behind the scenes and on the front lines within the medical school and the university to promote the nurse practitioner concept, garner support from influential key figures, and minimize opposition whenever he heard of it or came upon it. He was a stalwart believer in the expansive but untapped capabilities of nurses. Further, he knew that changing how nurses and doctors related to each other was essential to improving health care services. His contagious enthusiasm was, no doubt, a factor in convincing these seven nurses to jump on board that day.

Lucy Conant had come to UNC as a new dean with a relentless commitment to the nurse practitioner concept. She had endorsed the notion in 1965 when Loretta Ford started a Pediatric Nurse Practitioner (PNP) Program in Colorado. According to Conant, "My experience in public health nursing, my contact with nurse-midwives at Yale and in England, and particularly my experience as a district nurse in Cornwall, England, all had convinced me that there was a needed and viable role expansion for nurses."[4]

When Conant came to UNC for her initial visit as a candidate for the deanship, she learned, to her surprise—and delight—that Ike (Isaac) Taylor, dean of the medical school, shared similar views about nurses expanding their role and areas of responsibility. On her initial visit and subsequent visits, she found other kindred souls.[5] UNC was the place for her, and so in 1968, Conant became the second dean of the School of Nursing. She then spent the next two years preparing for this day. She somehow found a way—despite resistance from all but a few nursing faculty—to support and begin the Nurse Practitioner Program in the School of Nursing. This program was her baby! In her mind, it was going to happen and succeed or else. Since Conant was not bent on formalities—she was always Lucy, not Dean Conant—she easily conveyed a sense of camaraderie with the first seven nurses.

As Betty Compton introduced herself, she said she was not sure this was for her, but she was ready to take the risk. Dr. Pickard had made about three or four trips to talk to her about the program. By her recollection, he definitively asked her to join the program around early August; classes were to start the first week in September. She had no idea whether it was the right thing to do or not, but her intuition told her it was. So she hustled to arrange childcare and get recommendations for acceptance to the program.

Evelyn Aabel, Phoebe Hood, Ruth Efird, and Margaret Wilkman may have been acquainted or heard of each other; they certainly were not new to the campus. They all had been students in the School of Public Health at the same time. Wilkman had just finished coursework for her Master of Public Health (MPH) degree in the School of Public Health, across the street and within sight of Carrington Hall. As part of her studies, she worked with Glenn Pickard in the continuing care clinic at North Carolina Memorial Hospital, helping to identify information that would be important to include in a nurse practitioner curriculum. Wilkman also worked with the team that completed the *Prospect Hill Study*[6]—a study of health care needs in a small rural community in northern Orange County, North Carolina. The results were instrumental in identifying health care needs in rural communities.

Margaret Dolan, a national figure in public health, a nursing professor in the School of Public Health (SPH), and a strong supporter of the nurse practitioner concept, influenced Ruth Efird to "look into the new program in the School of Nursing." Efird was just finishing her MPH in nursing supervision when Dolan discussed the new program with her, just as she had done with Margaret Wilkman. They both knew it was a great opportunity. Other faculty in the SPH's Department of Maternal–Child Health encouraged Phoebe Hood, who had just finished her MPH in maternal–child health. The clinical nature of the Nurse Practitioner Program enticed Hood.

Evelyn Aabel was also a graduate of the master's program in maternal–child health from the School of Public Health. She had commented to Professor Seigel, a physician with an MPH and chair of the department, that she felt there was too little emphasis in the program on pediatric health—her primary interest. Seigel agreed, and he arranged for her to attend the Pediatric Nurse Practitioner Program in Denver, Colorado. She finished that program in the summer of 1970, and upon her return to Chapel Hill was asked to teach some of the child development content in the pilot Family Nurse Practitioner Program—which she did. At the same time, she enrolled in the program to add the "family" piece to augment her pediatric training.

The newly formed Orange–Chatham Comprehensive Health Services (OCCHS) Program, a partnership effort between the local Community Action Agency (CAA) and the university, was organized to develop clinics serving Orange and Chatham counties, bringing needed health care services to nearby rural areas. Community Action Agencies were a result of President Johnson's "War on Poverty" and the sweeping legislation enacted in 1964. A White House Office of Economic Opportunity administered federal funds to local Community Action Agencies. "The CAAs were charged with mobilizing local resources for a comprehensive attack on poverty by providing new services to the poor; coordinating all federal, state, and local programs dealing with the poor; and promoting institutional change in the interests of the poor."[7]

Mr. Paul Alston, director of the Orange–Chatham CAA, worked to develop health care services that would serve the rural poor in Orange and Chatham counties, and he simultaneously used the vehicle of an organized health care program to provide job opportunities for the poor in his area as well.

Alston particularly wanted to find nurses local to the communities the program would serve, so the CAA staff canvassed community leaders to identify qualified nurses. Since the majority of those living in poverty in the rural areas of Orange and Chatham counties were people of color, Alston, not having much time for student recruitment for the fall program, took it upon himself to find at least one nurse of color for the pilot program. He used his network of alumni from North Carolina Agricultural and Technical State University (NCA&T), a historically black university since 1891, to find nurses of color. He was fortunate to be referred to Glenda Hargraves, a nurse well-known in the community.

She had a newborn and could not be ready for the pilot program—but she said to him, please consider me for the program next year. I will be ready then! Hargraves, in turn, suggested another nurse in the community, Sandra Hogan. Hogan's child was now two years old, and she was ready to return to work. Her discussions with Alston, the clinical nature of the program, and direct contact with patients enticed Hogan to join the new program. Thus, the pilot program of seven included one nurse of color.

June Baise, from rural Walstonburg, in the eastern part of the state, was recruited by the community board responsible for planning and overseeing a new clinic in Walstonburg. She also was a known and trusted nurse from the area. After completing the program, Baise would return to Walstonburg and the new clinic being built there. The other six nurses would ultimately go to OCCHS clinics.

Their sense of what it had taken to get to this day was sketchy for those students in the pilot class. OCCHS, CAA, and OEO were not part of their professional vernacular. However, they knew there would be new clinics in their local areas to which they would return. They had no clear idea about the funding for the program or the source of their stipends; they assumed the university—a most reasonable assumption as their financial support came to them via the School of Nursing, even though originally from OCCHS. They had heard about this new program within only months of its beginning, yet they were willing to change course in their careers and seize what they sensed as a great opportunity.

It should be no surprise that five of the first seven nurse practitioner students came to the program with a public health background—both by experience and education. In their public health practice, they were often the sole resource for people living in rural and impoverished areas. They had to function independently. They often had to make diagnoses—although they would never have used that language of medical practice to describe what they did. But circumstances in their practice dictated that they do more than was authorized. They joined the nurse practitioner movement because they thought that the educational program would give them needed additional knowledge and skills, and more importantly, that such training would legitimize what they were already doing. For public health nurses, the Nurse Practitioner Program was highly valued and sought out.

Faculty in the School of Public Health, particularly those in the Departments of Maternal–Child Health, Public Health Nursing, and Health Policy and Administration, were aware of the acute challenges faced by local health departments, often the only source of health care for the poor and underserved in the state. They also knew local health departments struggled to find physician volunteers for their maternal and well-child clinics. Furthermore, nurses staffing those clinics had few referral sources. The same was true for the public health nurses in the field making home visits; they were limited by having few available referral sources and by uninsured patients' inability to pay private practice physicians. In the public health faculty's opinion, nurse practitioners could mitigate some of the challenges faced by local health departments. They saw the nurse practitioner as a natural extension of public health nursing, so they encouraged some of their students to enroll in the Family Nurse Practitioner Program.

We will return to this "First Day" of the new Family Nurse Practitioner Program, and to the early nurse practitioner graduates in subsequent chapters. While it is historic to mark September 1970 as the start of the first nurse practitioner program in North Carolina, it is equally important to ask how this first day came about. Many people had a hand in making the NP role and movement in North Carolina successful. Anyone who was intimately involved in the early years would say it was the result of the efforts of many. No one person can lay claim to formulating the concept of the NP. As with most innovations, the seed is planted many years earlier, from different visions and in different versions. New ideas build on past ones. Many factors, pressures, and experimentation with nursing roles contributed to the development of the nurse practitioner movement.

In North Carolina, a well-coordinated network orchestrated the political maneuvering it took to secure acceptance of NPs—by navigating, negotiating, and scheming within the university; within the legislature and state government; within and between organized medical and nursing organizations; and within and between local communities. This network extended the nurse practitioner movement from one that not only changed and enlarged the scope of nursing practice but also included a movement that changed health care delivery across the state of North Carolina. The nurse practitioner movement in North Carolina ushered in "a new order of things" to the practice of nursing and to the state's health care services for all its citizens.

In the next few chapters, we will go back to the sixties and examine the various ways nurses and physicians in the state and throughout the country began to experiment with new roles for nurses. We will show how the lack of available and accessible health care in the 1960s, particularly in rural areas, became a contributing factor in the development of the nurse practitioner movement. A close look at three North Carolina communities will highlight the struggles confronting individual rural communities as their leaders tried to solve what they each saw as their very own singular health care crisis. We will then return to the university's response to the articulated needs of rural communities and its leading role in the nurse practitioner movement in North Carolina.

As with most new ideas, it started before it started.

ADDENDA

Lead Allies toward a New Order of Things: A Closer Look

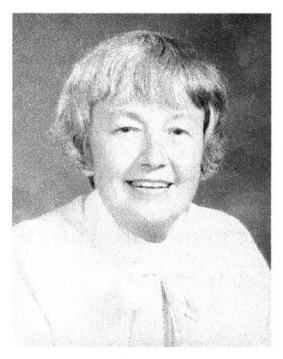

Lucy Houghton Conant, RN, PhD (1926–91), the second dean of the School of Nursing at the University of North Carolina at Chapel Hill, served as dean for seven years from 1968 to 1975.

During the summer before her final year at Radcliffe College, Conant spent a summer with the Frontier Nursing Service (FNS) in Kentucky as a "mounted carrier." What started out as an adventure became an eye-opening awareness for her about the poverty-stricken health and living conditions in rural Appalachia. Observing the FNS nurse-midwives at work sparked her interest in nursing.

Several years later, after earning her Master of Science in Nursing degree from Yale University, Conant's first job was as a visiting nurse for the County Health Department in Ann Arbor, Michigan. She told her brother that working as a visiting nurse was very different from working as a nurse in a hospital. "She was strictly on her own dealing with the practicalities of nursing in a variety of homes and personal situations."[8] After three years in Michigan, she wanted to experience for herself how nurses in England practiced. For a year, she worked as a district nurse in Cornwall, England, cementing her interest in public health.

She returned home and completed her MPH at Harvard University School of Public Health in 1957. Seven years later she finished her PhD in sociology at Yale University. Not surprisingly, her dissertation study examined nurse–patient relationships during home visits, and she continued to address issues in public health nursing. She was well primed to advocate for a greatly expanded role for nurses. Her interests and the goals of the University of North Carolina were a perfect match. Her background and experiences provided a strong platform for her to take on the challenge of starting the first family nurse practitioner program in North Carolina.

When Conant arrived in Chapel Hill in 1968, she also had another agenda—hiring the first School of Nursing black faculty member. A year later, she had recruited Carol Fray from Cornell University, the first faculty of color in the School of Nursing. No one was opposed to this idea. But Conant was the first to actively seek a black faculty member. This achievement was characteristic of Conant's sharply directed determination.

Those of us who worked with Conant found her to be affable while simultaneously serious about keeping focused on the goal. Her laugh was genuine and spontaneous, and not withheld when appropriate. She was warm, hospitable, informal, yet personally reserved. A classmate described her as "always herself, full of good will, gracious with a natural charm" and, as importantly, "soft but strong when the situation called for great strength."[9] She demonstrated that strength and good will for seven years as she pushed forward with the state's nurse practitioner movement. At her final graduation address in 1975, she stated her belief that "the expanded roles of nurses in 1975 will undoubtedly be the traditional roles of 2000."[10]

In 1975, Yale University School of Nursing presented Conant with a Distinguished Alumnae Award. Its citation reads, in part: "Always combining serious thought with laughter, she exhibits those qualities necessary for a craftsman in the art of nursing and a scholar of its science."[11] That same year as Conant was leaving Chapel Hill, she said it was time for her to pursue another "agenda for living." She yearned for the lush green pastures of western Massachusetts. And her farm—tending to it, putting her fingers in the soil, raising animals. Little did she know that she would have only a mere sixteen years more to pursue her second agenda for living.

Most of us who worked with Conant did not know of her personal writings, nor of her poetry. One poem written in the fall of 1974, just about the time she would have made known her decision not to seek a second term as dean, reveals much about her life beliefs.[12]

Immortality? Is it for real?
Let's count the things that last
The trees that you plant, the children you raise,
The deeds that you do, the words that you write,
The houses you build, the friendships you keep,
The kids that you teach, the music you make.
In living your life, you make your own world
That extends beyond you and past you
Into the future.
And, if God willing, there is more than all that,
Then your world of today is your world of tomorrow
And the future is now.

L.H.C.

Fall, 1974

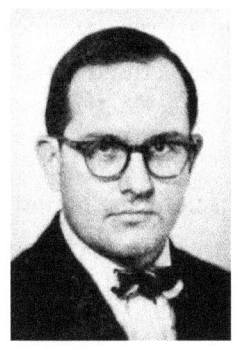

C. Glenn Pickard, Jr., MD (1936–2022), was, as the saying goes, "Tar Heel born, and Tar Heel bred." In his warm, friendly, and open manner (belied by his official photo here), he met and talked easily and respectfully with all he met, regardless of their station in life. When called on to resolve a difficult or disrupting situation involving rural local physicians and their concerns about nurse practitioners, his Carolina-bred manners, his good-natured, good-humored, and personable style, and his professional integrity and expertise helped him gain the acceptance and trust of local rural physicians.

Pickard received his undergraduate and medical degrees from the University of North Carolina at Chapel Hill and finished his internship at Columbia University. After a tour of duty in the U.S. Navy, Pickard returned to UNC for a residency in internal medicine, where in the continuing care clinic his ideas about the importance of nurses in health care delivery were clearly defined.

Pickard valued and respected nurses for their contributions to patient care services, and he knew they were capable of even more. Firmly convinced that the nurse practitioner role was a natural progression to advanced practice, he never faltered in this belief. All the nurse practitioners he taught remember his challenging them to explore and think further—without intimidation. Each one felt he was there for them alone, pushing and nudging until they believed in themselves. He took great pride in watching nurse practitioners grow in knowledge and self-confidence.

Pickard had a deep sense of social responsibility both for his own patients' personal health care and in the aggregate, for all the underserved in North Carolina. And knowing and loving North Carolina as he did, he knew the state and the health care system needed to do better for its mostly rural citizens. Nurse practitioners and rural primary care became his two top professional causes, for which he was an ardent crusader and unrivaled ambassador.

Pickard and Lucy H. Conant each held a love of the land, rivers, sea, and life outdoors close to their hearts—although that is not what bound them together. Their passion and dedication to elevating the practice of nursing and the health of the state's citizens bonded them in close collaboration for many years.

Pickard's love of the land started when he was young, exploring the forests and streams of the western Carolina mountains where he grew up. While working with nurse practitioners, he befriended a North Carolina

Cherokee Indian medicine man, Hawk Littlejohn. Pickard and Little-john hiked the mountains together, where Littlejohn taught Pickard about native plants and their use by medicine men. Often Pickard was able to link those native plants with derivatives used in modern pharmaceuticals. When in western North Carolina, he was never without a fly rod—just in case there was an opportune moment to cast his fly in a quiet, isolated mountain stream. He also learned to love the sea—the Atlantic at the far eastern end of the state—and he especially relished fishing off the coastal shore from remote and isolated barrier islands. Glenn Pickard was an outdoorsman dedicated to preserving and sustainably enjoying North Carolina's natural resources.

CHAPTER THREE

It Started Before It Started

A light bulb is turned on. A new idea, in similar fashion, flashes "on" in the mind. Rarely, however, does a new idea, a new way of doing emerge from the shadows clear and fully defined at the flip of a switch. Most innovations and ways of thinking are grounded in previous ways of thinking and/or doing. But incrementally over time, innovations are modified. That tinkering with accepted ways of thinking and doing gradually leads to what is called another innovation—something that looks different, is described differently, and, importantly, is given a new name. And again, in time and through various tweaks and iterations, that subsequent innovation becomes the accepted way of thinking and doing. This iterative process is as true for the idea of the nurse practitioner as it is for other innovations.

The idea of the nurse practitioner became something that looked different, was described differently, and was given a new name—and thus, it was an innovation when initially conceptualized in the mid-sixties and early seventies. Nurses and doctors,[1] at their core, are motivated to help people get well and to relieve their suffering; these motivations are central to who they are. Each health profession has a distinct role to play in achieving optimal health for patients, and each also has roles in common. Whenever something interferes with their ability to care for their patients, such as shortages or lack of access to or availability of services, they find ways to circumvent those barriers. They sometimes even push the boundaries of the law to do so, edging into territory that is not legitimized. And they experiment with new ways of doing. This was true when coronary care units emerged with nurses taking on added patient care responsibilities and was also true with the beginning of nurse practitioners as a newly defined nursing role.

Some of the experiments that helped form the core idea of the nurse practitioner are described below. They show us that the push to recognize the latent or underutilized talents and skills of nurses by enlarging their responsibilities and relying more on their clinical expertise had been going on well before the nurse practitioner movement began. The nurse practitioner movement took the results of these early demonstrations to their natural conclusion, and in doing so took a giant step forward in the clinical practice of nurses, well beyond the traditional role of nurses within the health care delivery system.

THE SIXTIES: CONTEXT OF THE TIMES

The Social Context

Social turbulence characterized the 1960s. The "sit-in" by young black men at Woolworth's lunch counter in Greensboro, North Carolina, set a pattern for nonviolent civil disobedience at the beginning of the decade, and the beginning of the civil rights movement. In the mid-sixties, the National Organization for Women was born after women concluded that polite petitions would not substantially advance their goal of equal rights with those of men. The Vietnam War bitterly divided Americans, with massive protests throughout the country. Many young Americans saw their friends lost to a needless war; some today continue to see the effects of this war among their parents' and grandparents' suffering, particularly from the devastating consequences of breathing and handling deadly chemicals like Agent Orange in that war. In the latter half of the decade, marches on Washington and protests across the country were frequent. The civil rights movement gained force and continued, sometimes violently, through the decade and on.

Every decade has its signature moments of shock and dismay, and the sixties were no different. Americans experienced remarkable highs and lows during the period. With horror, the nation watched a beloved young president, John F. Kennedy, being assassinated in November 1963. Almost five years later, the influential civil rights leader Dr. Martin Luther King, Jr., was gunned down, and a mere two months after that, another promising national leader, Robert F. Kennedy, was slain while campaigning for office in June 1968.

President Lyndon B. Johnson had come into office amidst much uncertainty. But within a year, he declared a "war on poverty," and quickly expanded his agenda into far-reaching programs for education, community development, and health care. The era of "The Great Society" was launched, with new national programs directed toward bettering the lives of disadvantaged Americans. By the end of the 1960s, the nation watched with exuberance as a man set foot on the moon for the first time in human history.

The Health Care System Context

The health care system did not escape the ethos of change during the decade either. President Lyndon Johnson's signature programs, Medicare and Medicaid, adopted by Congress on July 30, 1965, dramatically affected the health care system then and continue to do so today. In the sixties, aspiring presidential, congressional, and gubernatorial candidates raised the alarm over problems of health care access, availability, and quality. Primary care became a household term as local and national newspapers ran features about the nation's looming primary care crisis. The country's businessmen and labor leaders alike called for solutions.

Meanwhile, local communities watched the supply of health care services dwindle at the same time the postwar population exploded. The family doctor of generations past retired. Young doctors coming along to replace them were attracted instead to the technology, science, and specialties of burgeoning medical centers or were lured to lucrative practices in our growing suburbs. Rural areas were ignored, but soon it was clear that urban, inner-city areas were affected as well. The health care system was ripe for change.

Nationally, health care was declared, but not codified, a right for all citizens.[2] States and local communities had to address dire issues of nurse and physician shortages and the problems of access to and availability of health care services. Utilizing some of the previously unacknowledged abilities of nurses gained impetus in the mid-sixties as one solution to the shrinking availability of primary care services.

Others, especially nurses, saw the increased demand for services as an opportunity to strengthen and advance nurses' clinical role and decision-making authority in the health care system. Early endeavors involving experimentation with, and expansion of nursing roles contributed to the recognition of the underutilization of nurses. For instance, Montefiore Hospital in New York and the Los Angeles Health Department conducted demonstration projects in which nurses assumed almost total responsibility for uncomplicated obstetrical and pediatric care. Charles Lewis and Barbara Resnik experimented with a nurse clinic for chronic disease patients at the University of Kansas, and John Runyan experimented with nurse-run neighborhood clinics in Memphis. In 1965, Loretta Ford and Henry Silver introduced the Pediatric Nurse Practitioner Program at the University of Colorado.[3]

HEALTH CARE IN NORTH CAROLINA

As the nation began to address long-standing problems of access to and availability of health care, so did North Carolina. North Carolina was experiencing a severe shortage of physicians and had been for some

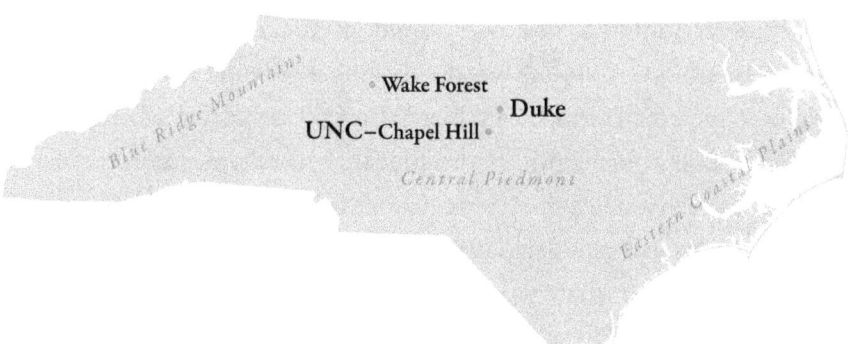

FIGURE 1. *Map of North Carolina regions, with three medical schools in the central Piedmont (not to scale).*

time. In 1967, North Carolina ranked forty-third among all states in the number of physicians per population.[4] Additionally, geographic maldistribution of physicians plagued North Carolina. In 1970, a cluster of seven counties in the northwestern corner of the state and eleven counties in the northeastern corner had half the number of physicians per population than the state average. In contrast, six counties in the central Piedmont section of the state had three times more physicians than the state average.[5] Not surprisingly, the central Piedmont was home to three medical schools.

Deficits in health care were not solely a local problem, however. A report submitted to the country's secretary of health, education, and welfare concluded that reform of the health care delivery system is expected by the American people, embraced by the health professions, and pledged as a goal by the president of the United States.[6] Like the nation, North Carolinians equated accessible and high-quality health care with a propitious physician-to-population ratio. Therefore, public demand for available and improved care took the form of calls for more physicians.

Even so, increasing the physician supply was a slow process: expanding medical school enrollments and establishing family practice residencies took a great deal of time and money, all of which was compounded by difficulties recruiting physicians to practice in rural and underserved areas. The fact that North Carolina was the nation's most rural state at the time, with few large urban areas, meant that the preponderance of efforts had to be devoted to enhancing primary health care in rural areas. State planning activities to increase health care services paralleled those on the national scene and spawned new legislation, new training programs for providers, new distribution strategies, and included a focus on grassroots health planning.

Some began to look to nurses as a focus of health care improvement, which led to the state's nurse practitioner movement. As early as the mid-1950s, Eugene Stead, MD, Thelma Ingles, RN, MSN, and Ruby Wilson, RN, EdD, attempted to formalize an advanced clinical nursing role by preparing master's degree nurse practitioners at Duke University. However, two denials of accreditation by the National League for Nursing forced Ingles, Wilson, and the School of Nursing to discontinue their innovative program. Stead turned his attention away from nursing, instead developing the nation's first physician assistant program in 1965.[7]

At the same time, the University of North Carolina (UNC) started the continuing care clinic where nurses took prime responsibility for following and managing patients with chronic diseases, which became a precursor to the Nurse Practitioner Program at UNC. In these early demonstrations, both at UNC and across the country, nurses ably demonstrated their advanced clinical knowledge and increased decision-making ability. Their competence gave credibility and impetus to what would become the nurse practitioner movement.

Pickard[8] traces North Carolina's nurse practitioner movement back to World War II. North Carolina was the state with the highest rejection rate for the draft during WWII. Black North Carolinians were rejected at a higher rate than white men; 61 percent of African American men were rejected while 40 percent of white men were rejected. Poor health status was the primary reason for these rejections. Embarrassment over the state's ranking as the state with the highest draft rejection rate led to North Carolina's statewide campaign after the war, dubbed the "Good Health Program."[9] North Carolina's "health" problem had to be solved by North Carolina. The governor and legislature took the issue of its citizenry's poor health status seriously and committed the state's treasury to the health improvement of North Carolinians by establishing the North Carolina Medical Care Commission of the Department of Health and Human Services in 1945.[10] Soon thereafter, in 1949, the legislature authorized new schools of nursing and dentistry and expansion of the University of North Carolina at Chapel Hill (UNC) medical school from a two-year to a four-year school. These new schools, along with the existing schools of pharmacy and public health, formed the Health Affairs Division of the University of North Carolina at Chapel Hill.

The legislative intent was broad, intending to provide needed health practitioners for the state as well as for all the university schools to provide needed services to improve the health of North Carolinians. Never again did North Carolina want to hold such a "first-place" ranking among other states in the country! As told by Glenn Pickard,[11] Dr. W. Reece Berryhill—dean of the medical school at the time—did not focus his recruitment of faculty solely on traditional biomolecular scientists. He also brought in some of the gurus who were thinking differently about health care delivery systems, such as Kerr White and William L. Fleming, and some younger activists such as Frank T. Williams and Robert R. Huntley.[12] White and Williams, along with epidemiologist Bernard Greenberg, wrote the classic paper, "The Ecology of Medical Care," in which they challenged health professional schools to give primary care research and teaching the same priority that had been accorded to research in the fundamental mechanisms of pathologic processes. They further noted that if only one adult out of one thousand per month was

referred to a university medical center and only five adults per one thousand per month was referred to another physician for consultation, students at university medical centers were not learning about the common
problems of health and illness experienced by people in communities
outside of the medical center.[13]

According to Pickard, the Berryhill recruits "set in place in this institution [UNC's medical school and hospital] the beginnings of a series
of programs that initially were very high in the institution's priorities.
For example, when they were organizing their outpatient clinic, this
institution absolutely refused to organize it along disciplinary [specialty]
lines."[14] This change in thinking led to a series of iterations in outpatient
care delivery that focused on providing primary care services, although
not called such at the time, rather than highly focused specialist care.

Over time, however, these efforts faltered as the medical and surgical
power brokers increasingly carved out their own disciplinary and subspe-
cialty clinics. Once the institution became more and more oriented to
providing specialty care, less and less primary care was available at UNC.
Many residents of the town of Chapel Hill had always looked to the
university for their medical care, but as the town grew, the primary care
system did not. The same was true for the adjacent town of Carrboro, the
small nearby town of Hillsborough, and rural areas in Orange County to
the north and in Chatham County to the south of Chapel Hill. Compounding this move to specialty-oriented care, the traditional general
practitioner was disappearing. Where there had been several local doctors, by the '60s there were few to none. Locals who needed care flooded
the UNC clinics—which were incapable of handling all the demand for
primary care. Despite the seeming reversal of emphasis though, a few
contrarians remained committed to providing comprehensive primary
care, in what was called the "general clinic" and subsequently the "continuing care clinic."

THE CONTINUING CARE CLINIC EXPERIMENT

By 1965, James (Jim) Bryan, II, Frank Williams, and Robert (Bob) Huntley were still struggling to organize a primary care model in the "midst of what, at that point, had become a completely tertiary care subspecialty-oriented hospital."[15] Glenn Pickard returned to UNC in 1965 and joined Bryan, Williams, and Huntley in their pursuit of a better model of care. The in-hospital/out-of-hospital, primary clinical and coordinator nurse was a central figure in this clinic—which was dubbed "the continuing care clinic."

Patients coming to the continuing care clinic did not need a referral from another doctor; they were coming for ongoing primary care, not for consultation with a specialist. A few physicians developed mechanisms to identify those coming to the UNC clinics who needed primary care, as opposed to consultative care, and a process of directing them to the continuing care team—an interdisciplinary team of doctors, nurses,[16] and social workers. After their medical assessment, Mary Cochran, the full-time nurse in the clinic, became their caretaker. She alternated days when she was in the clinic and when she made home visits. Betty West, a School of nursing faculty member with a joint appointment at the Chatham County[17] Health Department in Pittsboro, joined the continuing care team. Bryan and Pickard would refer patients to West, asking her to follow patients and report back if they ran into trouble. Often West called one or the other of these physicians to request prescriptions or other care modalities, or she would call to make an appointment for a patient she thought needed to see one of the physicians.[18]

Physicians in the continuing care clinic began to take notice of public health nurses. They soon discovered that public health nurses were already intervening, through public health department clinics for women and children and through home visiting to patients of all ages, and by so doing they were alleviating the gaps in health care access and availability.

They also learned that health care and healing does not always occur between the doctor and patient in the confines of the clinic exam room. The "doctor appointment" is merely a snapshot in a patient's experience of an illness or chronic condition. The physicians in the continuing care clinic quickly realized that they would know how a patient was doing primarily when a public health nurse called to report a problem or the need for an intervention.

At the same time, the continuing care team increasingly became aware of all that a nurse could do—in and out of the clinic. In response, they began teaching nurses more in terms of traditional medical assessment. Some School of Nursing faculty began to work with the physicians in the clinic, leading the way for clinical experiences for graduate nursing students. The doctors themselves began to appreciate the benefits of having nurses and social workers more involved in the care of patients. They also began to see that in terms of primary care, nurses could do much more as well as take on more responsibility. In these seminal ways the continuing care clinic "experiment" was foundational to UNC's Nurse Practitioner Program.

As crucial as the UNC continuing care clinic demonstration was to North Carolina's nurse practitioner development, there were similar developments across the country. Reports of these demonstrations in the mid to late sixties began to filter into the professional literature. The first report by Ford and Silver turned everyone's attention to what we now know as the pediatric nurse practitioner. Lewis and Resnik were the first to publish study results about nurses in expanded roles at the University of Kansas Medical Center clinics.[19] Other reports slowly followed.[20] In the sixties, however, there was no internet, email, or texting. The professional print literature lagged behind actual time by a year or two. Information about what others might be doing across the country relied on professional conferences, and, as importantly, word of mouth among colleagues scattered across the country. But even without the modern means of communication available today, those rare spirits trying something different managed to find each other—often across many miles.

Not only were a few physicians and nurses determined to maintain a primary care presence within the expanding specialization of the growing Medical Center at UNC. Local communities struggled as well, many trying to find ways to replace the family doctor who was no longer a leading presence in these communities. Three rural North Carolina communities exemplified rural communities of the 1960s. As importantly, community leaders tried to solve their own health care problems; some made their needs known to the university. Their pleas for help found their way to those trying to forge a place in the system for continuing comprehensive care, or what we would today call primary care.

The efforts of local community leaders, along with the continuing care clinic experiment, became a force and a model for the development of the nurse practitioner movement in North Carolina. Although not wholeheartedly accepted by all nurses and physicians, many endorsed nurse practitioners as one solution to the problems confronting our ailing health care system. In its early formative stages, some saw nurse practitioners simply as a temporary solution to the physician shortage and lack of primary care services, particularly in rural and other underserved areas. But those involved in the nurse practitioner movement saw it as a reform movement, and to some it was even a revolution. They saw nurse practitioners as strengthening and elevating the practice of nursing within the health care community and with patients and consumers. They did not see nurse practitioners as "doctor alternatives" but instead saw them as a new way, a preferable way of providing primary health care services. To them, the nurse practitioner role was a natural evolution of the practice of professional nurses.

CHAPTER FOUR

Three Community Prototypes

Three North Carolina communities exemplified the health care problems faced by many rural communities throughout the state. Like other eastern coastal states, North Carolina is divided into three north–south regions. Mountains and foothills distinguish the western part of the state, whereas coastal plains and marshes characterize the east. The central portion of the state, known as the Piedmont, is marked by lush rolling hills. Despite their disparate geography and varying social and economic characteristics, a small local community in each of the three regions of North Carolina faced a similar dilemma: they lacked health care services. Each approached their problem differently, but they all arrived at a comparable solution. Although they took slightly different paths to their solutions, all three developed a health system that relied on the use of nurse practitioners. Each of these communities developed the first exemplary nurse practitioner–staffed community clinic in their part of the state. And all three clinics are still open and serving the public today in 2022.

PROSPECT HILL: CENTRAL PIEDMONT

In the late sixties, Prospect Hill was a community not unlike many rural areas across the country before the 1960s: most residents enjoyed a stable source of health care, namely a dedicated private family physician. In the mid-sixties, however, this security was threatened. Many country and

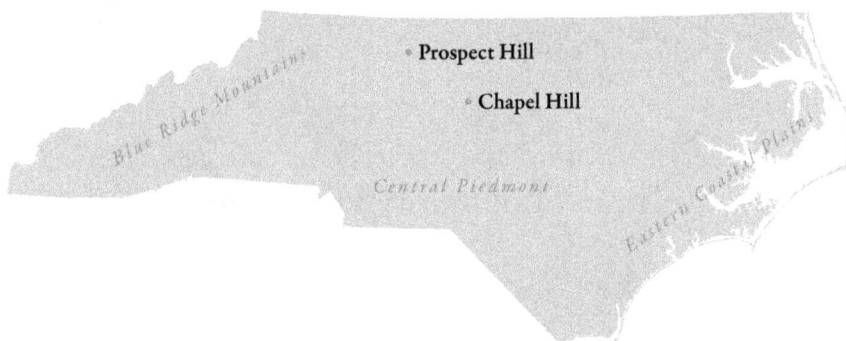

FIGURE 2. *Map of North Carolina regions, UNC-Chapel Hill, and the rural town of Prospect Hill (not to scale).*

family doctors were nearing retirement, and there were no replacements as new physicians were attracted to practices in medical centers and urban areas. The health care problems Prospect Hill residents faced then were similar to those of many other small communities. Yet Prospect Hill was unique in the dedication and persistence among interested residents and leaders as they attempted to solve their health care problem.

Prospect Hill of the sixties was a crossroads community where the Warren name figures prominently in its history. Mrs. Geneva Warren, a community leader, played a central role in the development of a new system of health care in Prospect Hill during the sixties. Geneva's husband, Joseph Warren, also a community leader and highly respected local merchant, had been a representative in the state legislature for several terms immediately preceding his untimely death in 1966. However, the impetus to find a new doctor starts with "Doc" Warren, the cousin of Geneva's late husband, Joseph.

Doc Warren: A Loyal Family Doctor

"Doc Warren," Dr. R. F. Warren, was a familiar name in the Prospect Hill community, a man loved and revered. He knew all the people of the area—their families, their grandparents, and their children. "Doc" provided emotional counsel as well as medical care to the entire community. At a time when black and white communities were separate, he provided care to both alike. He expressed his dedication to the people of the Prospect Hill area in many ways. Ability to pay was never a consideration. In fact, most of the time, he didn't even keep track of who owed him.[1] Shortly before Doc Warren died in 1958, anticipating retirement, he approached several community leaders about the need to recruit another physician to the area. His daughter, a physician, like many other physicians of the time, had found her niche at the University of North Carolina at Chapel Hill (UNC), forty-plus miles away, with no quick route as travel was via 1960s-era two-lane secondary roads. Doc Warren's daughter was not interested in returning to live or practice in Prospect Hill and following in her father's footsteps. Since there was no one else in the community who could assume his role, he saw the urgent need to recruit a physician, for, in his absence, the region would be without any source of health care.

On Saturday, May 11, 1957, a small group of community leaders from religious and civic organizations, as well as several representatives from adjoining communities, met to discuss the possibility of building a health clinic at Prospect Hill.[2] The community had sought to attract another physician but to no avail. Perhaps a new clinic building would provide the enticement needed to recruit a physician, so the community embarked on a fundraising campaign to build a new clinic building. Black leaders were enlisted to raise funds for the new clinic from their communities and church groups, as they too would be beneficiaries of care from a new doctor replacing Doc Warren.

The community leaders intended that the collective community effort and the clinic building would serve to honor Doc Warren's service of forty-eight years. The fundraising drive was highly successful, with virtually every resident of the community contributing some amount for the clinic building, from one dollar to a few hundred dollars. Unfortunately, Doc Warren died in 1958, unable to witness the completion of the building and its dedication as a memorial to him. The clinic building was eventually completed in 1961, using borrowed funds to supplement the money donated by residents. Yet no physician had been attracted to the community. On several occasions, community groups through Mrs. Geneva Warren had approached the UNC medical school for assistance, but although they found sympathetic ears, there were no immediate takers of the offer.

Geneva Warren: A Most Gracious Political Activist

Several years later, in 1967, as the new clinic building still sat idle, without a physician, a loan on the building for approximately five thousand dollars came due. Mrs. Warren summoned a few community leaders to meet one Sunday morning in August. They were clearly not ready to see foreclosure on the clinic building and its conversion to a barbershop, beauty shop, or some other business. The clinic was, after all, not only an attractive means for recruiting a new physician—so they thought—but also a memorial to Doc Warren, and they were not ready to give up either intention. By that time, the local public that had held bake sales and "nickeled and dimed" to build the clinic had lost faith and interest. These community leaders decided that Sunday afternoon to pay off the loan on the clinic building, and each pledged eight hundred dollars to do it.

With no doctor in sight, Mrs. Geneva Warren asked the sponsors— the clinic noteholders—if she could contact Dr. Sarah Lou Warren, a physician at UNC and Doc Warren's daughter. She would inquire about the University of North Carolina medical school's interest in owning and/or operating the Prospect Hill clinic. An earlier plan for bringing some sort of health care involving the university had fizzled out, but perhaps Geneva Warren could rekindle the university's interest. During her discussions with Doc Warren's daughter at the School of Medicine, Mrs.

Warren saw that the possibility of health care in Prospect Hill was looking more promising. She was referred to the dean and subsequently to Dr. Glenn Pickard, the leading proponent of North Carolina's nurse practitioner movement.

Dr. Pickard was one of several young internists on the medical school faculty who experimented with new patterns for delivery of comprehensive health care and in educating nurses to participate more centrally in health care delivery to the underserved areas of predominantly rural North Carolina. Dr. Pickard had inherited the medical school's previous efforts, and he saw this moment of Mrs. Warren's contact as an opportunity to push his agenda for nurse practitioners. In her continuing discussions with Dr. Pickard, Mrs. Warren learned of the idea of nurse practitioners. The possibility of getting nurse practitioners to Prospect Hill kept the community's hopes alive. *aha!*

After a nine-year courtship, the university said yes in 1969. They would train nurse practitioners to staff the clinic. Ten years after constructing the new clinic building, the possibility of some health care was on the horizon.

From their first meeting in the summer of 1969, Dr. Pickard and Mrs. Warren stayed in contact throughout the fall of 1969 and spring of 1970. The Pickard–Warren partnership was fortuitous for both. Mrs. Warren found an advocate for rural primary care in Dr. Pickard. Dr. Pickard found an ally in Mrs. Warren, an influential partner with political connections who could help secure funding for the upstart Nurse Practitioner Program and clinic services in Prospect Hill.

Geneva Warren came to Prospect Hill in 1941 as an unmarried schoolteacher. She met and married Joseph H. Warren, a businessman, community leader, and member of the North Carolina State House for several terms before it became the House and Senate. During Joseph Warren's legislative service, Geneva and Joseph became good friends with the influential Scott family of neighboring Alamance County.[3] By the time Mr. Warren died, Senator Ralph Scott's family and the Warrens were close friends.

In the many conversations between Dr. Pickard and Mrs. Warren, Pickard often expressed his reservations about whether their ideas would come to fruition. According to Mrs. Warren,

> He didn't give me much reason to hope. But I said, "Well, I do. I don't claim to have many friends in the legislature, but my husband did, and he had friends who were very loyal to him, and he was loyal to them. And if that kind of thing makes any difference, if money from the legislature makes any difference, I'll work for it. I don't know if I'll have any success at all. I do not know, but I could try. But does this matter?" He said, "You betcha it does! It makes a lot of difference."[4]

Mrs. Warren went back again to talk with Pickard, asking if he had any written material she could use when she spoke to one of the Scotts. That request set off a slew of quite essential and influential letters—which got things moving in short order. On March 18, 1969, Dr. Pickard wrote to Mrs. Warren, sharing with her a budget request to fund the endeavors he and she had discussed. That was all she needed.

A month later, on April 14, 1969, Mrs. Geneva Warren sent a handwritten letter to Governor Robert W. Scott, telling him about this proposal and how she thought his "support would be a natural for the Scott family." Mrs. Warren also paid a visit to Senator Ralph H. Scott about the budget proposal. Senator Ralph Scott was the influential chairman of the Senate Finance Committee, and fortuitously he was also the uncle of Governor Robert Scott. Mrs. Warren's meeting with Senator Ralph Scott prompted a phone call from Senator Scott to Dean Taylor of the medical school. Shortly thereafter, one day during rounds, Dr. Pickard surprisingly found himself taking a phone call from Senator Ralph Scott about the program outlined in the medical school's budget request.

In the span of one month, Mrs. Warren's letter and visit to family friends who happened to be serving as governor and state senator brought to their attention a particular budget proposal that was a part of the entire university's budget proposal that year. Mrs. Warren's request was well timed and well received. A few weeks later, on May 2, 1969, Senator Ralph Scott informed the State Budget Officer by letter, copied to Mrs. Geneva Warren, that this budget request was something he was "vitally concerned about." And then on May 15, Governor Robert "Bob" Scott wrote to Mrs. Warren, saying that he had expressed his support for the budget request from the Division of Education and Research in Community Medical Care, a division in the School of Medicine. He assured her that the legislative leaders he had talked to informed him the request was still on the approved list. Shortly after the university's budget request had been approved, the dean's office of the medical school wrote to Senator Scott, thanking him for his help in securing the budget request and assuring him that the school would continue with the implementation of the programs authorized by the legislature.[5]

Although Mrs. Warren had told Dr. Pickard that she wasn't sure whether she would have any success in calling on her husband's friends, five months later it was clear that she did. She had simply never done anything like this before. Geneva Warren describes it this way:

Well, if you think I was scared to go see Glenn [Pickard], you should have seen me when I went to see Senator Scott. He had been a friend of the family when Joseph [Warren] died. He had come to Joseph's funeral but was unable to stay; he became so overcome with—we probably did look pretty pitiful with four children at their ages. Anyway, I went. I had never lobbied anybody about anything. I went into his office, and with his southern Alamance County drawl...he just absolutely made me feel so much more comfortable right away. I just told him what I wanted, and I said, "Now, I don't know, this may seem unlikely to you because we're such a small community and all, but we think we ought to give it a good try, at least do everything that we can, and then if it just won't work, we're satisfied. We'll be satisfied then to let it drop."

So he said—by the way, he was chairman of the Finance Committee for the Senate at that time, and his nephew was governor of North Carolina—Bob. So he said, "Well, I'll talk to the governor about it. Don't feel bad or apologize for coming and asking about it because most of the time, folks want something just for themselves, and you're wanting this for the community." He gave me a lot of reassurance, and I felt a little better about it.[6]

In discussing all of this, Geneva Warren frequently referred to loyalty and how important it was. She said, "The Scotts don't forget you. If you're their friend, they are your friend till death. And I just felt like I was being heard, and I couldn't believe it. That loyalty came from long ago." This would not be the last time Geneva Warren would use her connections to solve problems and mitigate opposition related to nurse practitioner practice. This also would not be the last time that loyalty, particularly among professional colleagues, would be consequential to the nurse practitioner movement's continuing progress.

Geneva Warren's nurturing of political connections, and sparingly using those connections only for important reasons, illustrates one way to successfully attain the attention and action from state legislators and elected officials. Mr. David Warren, unrelated to the Warrens of Prospect Hill, was an attorney with the UNC Institute of Government. The institute was established in 1932 to provide educational, advisory, and research support for local and state government officials.[7] David Warren worked with those involved in developing the Family Nurse Practitioner Program at UNC, providing guidance about the legal aspects of nurse practitioner practice. After many years of working with state legislators, David Warren believed that what it takes to get the attention of legislators is

> something you can't calculate. You can do all you want in academia [studying] and writing articles, or spend hours and days working through the state nurses association to develop a resolution or something, which will never be heard by the legislature until there's something else that causes the issue to be put on the front burner. Then the resolution from the state nurses association may be brought in, in testimony. But it usually is not going to be the initiating thing. It's going to be something more personal that initiates some legislative attention to a topic.[8]

When a citizen brings an important issue or problem to a senator or representative, the legislator usually pays attention and may investigate. The time for professionals to act is after a personal issue is brought forward. Professionals seeking some change or favorable legislative action can then step in to support and influence public discourse about a proposed legislative action. This is what Geneva Warren did: bring an important matter to a senator's attention. Then, and only then, could advocates within the university intervene and be heard.

We leave Prospect Hill for the moment, recognizing it as a community with needs for health care services, just like so many other rural communities, but also a community with a unique sense of leadership. For good reason, then, the first NP clinic in North Carolina opened there. We will return to their story.

WALSTONBURG: THE EASTERN COASTAL PLAINS

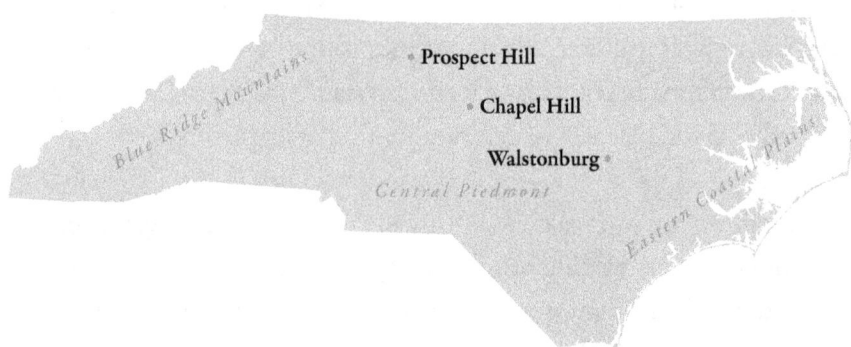

FIGURE 3. *Map of North Carolina regions, the university, and the rural towns of Prospect Hill and Walstonburg (not to scale).*

Walstonburg is Main Street America, a town of fewer than 200 residents, and no more than 1,200 additional residents in the surrounding countryside. Like other areas across North Carolina and the country, in 1968, its health care system was deteriorating because of the death of the country doctor and the flight of younger physicians to more urban areas. The development of Walstonburg's new health care system involved community leaders but was also closely linked to events at the University of North Carolina at Chapel Hill. Walstonburg's use of nurse practitioners came about by a combination of chance and opportunity, with a larger dose of the latter.

Cecil Sheps: A Public Health Advocate and Health Services Researcher

In 1969, Dr. Cecil Sheps came to the university as director of the newly funded Health Services Research Center (HSRC, a.k.a. the Center). As Sheps went about appointing staff and setting the direction of the Center, he and the staff identified two problems they were going to address. One was to "convert services to programs," Sheps's motto and now the Center's motto, and the second was to "solve problems of rural health care." He certainly was in an area where both endeavors were needed.

Very soon after arriving in North Carolina, Sheps was present at a community meeting one evening in late April 1969, in Wilson, North Carolina, a town near Walstonburg. As Cecil tells it, his presence there was related to his position as director of the HSRC.

> I was invited to a lot of places—because we [the Center] had a lot of money, and people thought all of their problems could be solved by that, and so on. I went to Wilson, North Carolina, to talk about the Center, and two men who were county commissioners of Greene County [Walstonburg] ...said to me, "Maybe you can help us find a new doctor."[9]

Sheps took advantage of the opportunity.

> Gently I moved them into a situation where I could say: look, you're never going to get a doctor—forget it.... But I said, I think we can do something that might be just as good, maybe better, and certainly permanent.[10]

Then Sheps explained his idea—a nurse practitioner clinic with physician backup from one of the nearby communities. His notion was an adapted version of the original pediatric nurse associate model developed by Ford and Silver[11] in Denver, Colorado. Sheps had learned about the Ford and Silver model before he came to North Carolina. He supported it and brought that support with him to North Carolina. He knew of the plans to begin a nurse practitioner training program in the School of Nursing, so he felt confident in continuing his discussions with the leaders in Greene County. A year later, in 1970, Jim Bernstein arrived in Chapel Hill—and Sheps "put him to work on Walstonburg, together with a nurse who was getting a PhD in the School of Public Health, Jessie Pergrin. Jessie and Jim, I put them both to work in Walstonburg."[12]

Jim Bernstein: The Man behind the Rural Health Scene

How did Bernstein, a New York City guy by birth, a Johns Hopkins graduate in political economy, a Peace Corps volunteer in Morocco, a master's graduate in hospital administration from a School of Public Health in the Midwest,[13] and an administrative resident in Cleveland, Ohio, get to Chapel Hill, North Carolina? James "Jim" Bernstein arrived in Chapel Hill by way of Santa Fe, New Mexico, where he had served as an administrator in the Indian Health Service, part of the Public Health Service, where he had been an officer since 1966.

While in Santa Fe, Bernstein became interested in community development, particularly in the area of community health care systems. Earlier he had served on the planning committee for a community-run nurse practitioner clinic in New Mexico. Bernstein, to use his words, was "revved up" by working with Dr. Robert Oseasohn, chairman of community medicine and epidemiology at the University of New Mexico. Oseasohn had provided training to a nurse, whom he described as a physician assistant, and with a federal grant started a clinic to provide primary care to a small town, Estancia, New Mexico, with backup from physicians in Albuquerque—mainly by telephone. It was this positive experience that shaped the focus of Bernstein's application for a fellowship in "Global Community Health" from the U.S. Public Health Service. The Public Health Service wanted "Global Fellows"—as they were known— to "bridge the gaps of our time by respecting tradition but refusing to be bound by it..., and to bring a sensitivity and commitment to alleviate the health problems of the community."[14] That fit Bernstein to a "T."

Bernstein submitted his Global Fellowship application, writing: "When I wrote my application in '69 for this fellowship, it was around using nurse practitioners and PAs in developing community-run clinics. That was specifically what I was going to do, in rural areas—a very specific application."[15] Global Fellows were free to decide where they would spend their three years of study, which usually included an advanced degree program. Jim began to ask around about a prominent place with an appropriate fit for his fellowship years.

Jim Bernstein had come to know Glenn Wilson while he was in Cleveland for his administrative residency. Mr. Wilson was vice president of the Kaiser Health Plan there for the Ohio region. Jim called Wilson, seeking his advice. At the time, Wilson was completing negotiations at UNC to become associate dean for community affairs of the School of Medicine. Jim was considering a couple of places, but Wilson told him that he needed to go to Chapel Hill, talk with Cecil Sheps, and to consider the School of Public Health.

So, Bernstein did just that. On his Chapel Hill visit, after he had spoken with several people, Sheps sent Bernstein to Wilson, North Carolina, to meet Dr. Edgar Beddingfield and later that night with a group of citizens from Greene County who wanted to build a health center. Afterward, Bernstein reflected on those meetings in his reporting to Sheps:

> Well, look, I'm down there talking to this guy Beddingfield and dah, dah, dah, dah, dah. Glenn Wilson and Cecil were like this then [two fingers held together], good buddies, because Glenn was the one who told me to see Cecil. Glenn hadn't gotten here yet. Glenn was just interviewing here, and he said, "Well, you got to come. This is the place to look." I…came down here right away and looked. It was just what I wanted to do. There it was. I don't know where Cecil got his ideas, and you guys [Freund and Booth] got your ideas. I know where I got mine, from [working in] Estancia and [from] Dick Smith.[16]

Walstonburg became Bernstein's fellowship work, supervised by Sheps. Bernstein felt strongly that his and the university's role should be one of providing technical assistance to the Walstonburg community. Bernstein, Pergrin, and Sheps helped the Walstonburg community organize itself, identify local leadership, and conduct a fundraising campaign. They helped establish a local committee that went to churches, community meetings, and door-to-door to collect money for a clinic building. The money they raised, together with a $30,000 grant Sheps had secured for Walstonburg from the Z. Smith Reynolds Foundation,[17] was put toward a clinic building.

The clinic and the services it would provide would be owned and run by a community board of directors, residents of the area. Bernstein worked intensively with the board to develop a health care service. Although the community had wanted initially to recruit a physician, they soon adopted the idea of a nurse practitioner clinic. The university would train a nurse practitioner for Walstonburg in its first class, along with those it would prepare for Prospect Hill.

Because of the distance between Walstonburg and the university in Chapel Hill, eighty-six miles and two hours by car, Sheps knew that the success of the Walstonburg clinic would be dependent on the support of a physician or a group of physicians nearby. Thus, while Walstonburg was raising funds and organizing its board of directors, Sheps sought the backing of a group of physicians in Wilson, a town eight miles from Walstonburg.

Sheps described a meeting he had had with the group. Sheps had already agreed to commit money from the Health Services Research Center to help Walstonburg start its clinic. It was natural that he also offer money to the Wilson physician group to provide backup services to the Walstonburg clinic. They said no, however. Sheps talked about the need for care and the problems of accessibility. They still declined, saying that patients eventually end up coming to their clinic anyway. Sheps continued to plead:

THREE COMMUNITY PROTOTYPES   53

I said, "You're the major resource in this part of the state, and the public expects you to be helpful." I couldn't change their minds about anything. I said, "If you do this in Walstonburg, and then another place, you'll be doing something that nobody else is doing." It did not make any difference.[18] *They said N.O.*

However, there was one physician in the group for whom the idea made sense—Edgar T. Beddingfield, Jr. Dr. Beddingfield spoke in favor of the group's involvement with Walstonburg. But being the most recent member to have joined the group practice, and as one of the few general practitioners among many specialists, he did not wield enough power to persuade the group.

After the meeting, Beddingfield told Sheps that he would provide the backup services for the Walstonburg clinic. A native of the area, he was committed to meeting the needs of fellow residents. He later enlisted another physician from the group, John McCain, to work with him and with the Walstonburg clinic.

The alliance between Beddingfield and the Walstonburg community was fortunate. It not only paved the way for Walstonburg to open its health clinic in 1973, but more importantly, it got Beddingfield involved with nurse practitioners. Even though Beddingfield was not influential with his physician group locally, he was a powerful medical statesman in the state medical society and the American Medical Association.

We will return to Walstonburg again, for the Walstonburg experience served as a testing ground to what would later become the North Carolina Rural Health Program, designed and directed by Jim Bernstein. And we will meet up with Ed Beddingfield again, as his support and political influence were crucial during challenging times in the early years of the nurse practitioner movement.

THE HOT SPRINGS SAGA: THE WESTERN MOUNTAINS

Mountain lore comes alive as one approaches Hot Springs, a rural mountain community. Although Hot Springs is only thirty miles west of Asheville, North Carolina, a sizable city by North Carolina standards even in the 1970s, it took sixty minutes by car to get from Asheville to Hot Springs along the curving, mountainous roads of the Smokies. From the two-lane state road, one turns onto a six-mile secondary road that curves around the winding French Broad River. The last curve into Hot Springs crosses the French Broad; there, nestled in the mountains, sits the scenic town.

Unlike Prospect Hill, Hot Springs is more than a crossroads. In 1970, it was a small town. In the 1940s, Hot Springs had thrived on tourism, and a grand hotel once anchored the town's economy. Hot Springs also had its general store, a few businesses that served the community, and a small manufacturing plant—closed as often as it was open. In the mid-1960s, the town attempted to renew itself, once again catering to the tourist trade—appealing especially to hikers, river runners in rafts and canoes, and backpackers.

Nurse practitioners came to Hot Springs in ways that differed from those of Prospect Hill and Walstonburg, too. Hot Springs did not have

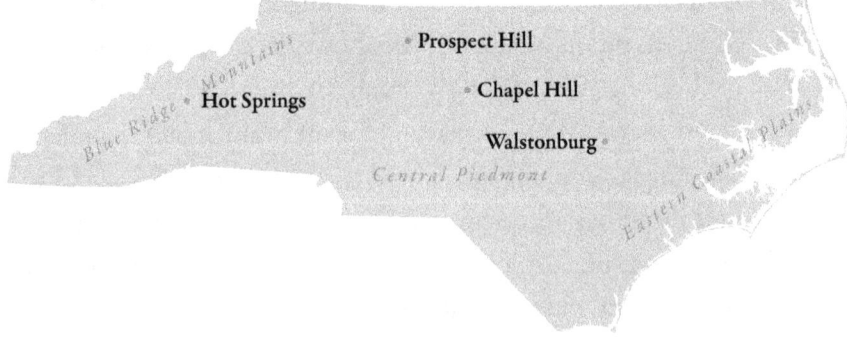

FIGURE 4. *Map of North Carolina regions, the university, and the rural towns of Prospect Hill, Walstonburg, and Hot Springs (not to scale).*

prominent families, influential community leaders, or a tradition of health care over generations that citizens wanted to sustain. The system of health care in Hot Springs grew out of the involvement of a social activist in the early '60s.

Linda Mashburn: A Public Health Nurse and Social Activist

Linda Mashburn was a committed, crusading young nurse who was influenced by the Frontier Nursing Service in Kentucky. She was a public health nurse in the broadest and best sense. Before coming to Hot Springs, she spent five years working for the Southern Regional Appalachian Commission and the United Presbyterian Church, in a job similar to serving as a domestic Peace Corps volunteer. While with the Southern Regional Appalachian Commission, Mashburn went from mountain community to mountain community, setting up health fairs to educate people on health, to provide a general assessment of their health status, and to arouse their awareness of health issues. Often, in the momentum of the fairs, other social and community issues were addressed. According to Mashburn,

> The primary goal of the church in the health fairs that I was involved in organizing was community organization.... Of course, health fairs were somewhat successful in terms of health education that took place in and around them, and some screening, or screenings, where that was possible and feasible.... But they saw the health fair as primarily a vehicle for getting people in a rural community that had no health services to begin talking about what their health needs were, to begin organizing around some of those needs, and figuring out ways to meet them.
>
> My primary work during the winter was following up on those health fairs and developing community leadership, ideas, and

enthusiasm that grew out of the successful event of the health fair—to build on it with other things…. We felt the health fair stimulated and encouraged community leadership in areas where there wasn't a lot of community leadership.[19]

Mashburn saw firsthand many of the problems arising from a lack of accessible and available health care. After five years of frustration at being able to deal only superficially with health issues and spending many miles on the road traveling to separate mountain communities, Mashburn felt ready to settle down to work more comprehensively on health issues. She had been to Hot Springs on several occasions with health fairs. She had gotten to know several of the community's leaders and saw Hot Springs as a potential place to develop her ideas. Several things attracted her to Hot Springs.

First, health care was the number one priority of the Hot Springs people. The community had a building the people refurbished—a cinder block building, empty for eight years with a caved-in roof, rented for one dollar from the owners. They renovated it for the first health fair in 1969, and it became the local center for health care. Second, there was a good community organizer, in Linda's own words,

a local person who could do a lot of community organizing for me or with me and who had sufficient knowledge of the leadership in that area to keep me out of some of the major pitfalls that are easy for an outsider to fall into. When you don't know the lay of [the] political land, and you don't know who's talking to whom and where the factions lie, it's easy to blunder about. He [Jerry Plemmons] had a lot of contacts and was neutral enough to demand respect from the various factions.[20]

A third attraction, strangely enough, was the relative isolation of Hot Springs, which precluded immediate major opposition from the local medical society.

> I had battled enough medical societies by then over health fairs, just getting permission to do a few heights and weights and blood pressures, you know—frivolous things like that. The commissioner of health of one state had called me up and threatened legal action against me. He declared he'd get an injunction on the health fair— all kinds of crazy things. We had to get legal counsel before I went ahead with the health fair in that state.[21]

Given the strengths that Mashburn saw in the Hot Springs community, she settled there and began to stimulate interest in her ideas for a health care system. Soon Mashburn, being the public health nurse she was, opened a clinic and started offering services herself.

> I moved to Hot Springs in January of '71. We opened the clinic with five hundred dollars, which the community raised, on May 1 in 1971. Everybody worked, at that point, on a stipend or very little. I don't think I pulled a salary for several months after that, but I did pay another volunteer nurse a little stipend, and we had two volunteer girls who were unemployed in the community—one was on welfare at the time—who volunteered their services. And then we paid our physician from Asheville something like a hundred dollars a day to come out. So, for the first several months, from at least May till September, we ran almost strictly on volunteer services. In September, I got a five-thousand-dollar grant from a foundation, so then we really did put people on a formal stipend—like a little payroll.[22]

Linda had learned a great deal from the Frontier Nursing Service, and in particular, from a little outpost community in Tennessee—Clairfield. Every outpost had a nurse with basic public health training and a nurse-midwife. She saw the kinds of standing orders and referral systems they used. And she observed the nurses in the clinics provide well childcare and treat minor health problems. From these experiences, she developed her notion of health services for rural mountain communities: "some combination of public health nursing in which there was heavy stress on education and prevention, along with acute and chronic treatment."[23] A year or so later, Linda learned of the Nurse Practitioner Program in Chapel Hill; she visited, and then her vision of the Hot Springs community health system expanded. She learned that nurse practitioners, with physician backup and consultation, could offer more services than she originally envisioned.

Because two neighboring communities were also in need of health care, she soon expanded her operation through a grant from the Z. Smith Reynolds Fund, which was followed by a larger grant from the Kate B. Reynolds Health Care Trust.[24] The Hot Springs community health system, including two satellite clinics, began. Mashburn recruited several trained nurse practitioners from other parts of the country and brought them to Hot Springs and the surrounding communities. At this time, she was also able to recruit a part-time physician.

Although town leaders were involved in the development of the Hot Springs health system, the community's role initially was primarily that of a supporter and assistant, following the lead of the social activist. Mashburn was not an original resident of the area. Yet these mountain communities, which tend to be closed-minded about new ideas from the outside, paradoxically accepted her proposals. Mashburn, and the professionals she recruited to Hot Springs, eventually assimilated into the community as part of the community's health system.

THE THREE COMMUNITY PROTOTYPES

The three community prototypes described above were like other small rural communities across the country in the problems they faced in the 1960s. An increasing demand for health care services, accentuated by the departure or retirement of the local family doctor just as new physicians set up group practices in more populated areas, resulted in a maldistribution of physicians; consequently, many smaller communities faced similar dilemmas. The fact that these three communities were rural does not necessarily make them distinct from urban communities regarding their health needs. Urban regions, particularly inner cities within large metropolitan urban areas, faced similar problems: physicians flocked to the suburbs and left inner cities without a source of health care.

Even before the mid-sixties, there had been various experiments with alternative delivery systems. The Frontier Nursing Service in eastern Kentucky had been in existence for some time and had recently expanded its services beyond midwifery in response to the need for primary care services in rural mountain communities. Linda Mashburn's experience with the Frontier Nursing Service, for example, shaped her views and ideas about the evolving health system in Hot Springs. Lewis and Resnick in Kansas, Loretta Ford and Henry Silver at the University of Colorado in Denver, Oseasohn in New Mexico, and others all called attention to the crisis in health care and the need for alternative care systems.

Initially, the search for health care solutions in local communities tended to focus on traditional answers: the doctor's office building that was supposed to attract a new doctor. This effort was usually followed by the formation of a board to spearhead the search for a new family doctor. The doctor quest sooner or later led to the medical schools, and, in North Carolina, that meant UNC. The community boards found or interested others in searching for logical answers, and they included academic health science schools, professional health care organizations, state and federal government agencies, and politicians. Thus, in many ways, the three communities' need for health care described above were more similar than unique. What they illustrate is that there was a need for health care services, there were problems to be addressed, and communities were struggling with these lacunae in various ways. Eventually, each of these communities adopted the nurse practitioner model to meet their needs.

Fifty years later and beyond, each of the three communities ended up as part of a thriving regional health care system. But the road from the 1970s to the 2020s was not always smooth. There were crises along the way that threatened the viability of not only each new community health care system, but nurse practitioners as well. We will revisit each of these communities to examine their struggles as an integral part of the development and evolution of the North Carolina nurse practitioner movement. In the beginning years of the nurse practitioner movement in North Carolina, unlike other early nurse practitioner programs, the university became partners with local community leaders in forging an effective and long-lasting local health care system.

It was an embarrassment that 40% of NC. ♂ flunked their physical for the draft in the 1940's.

ADDENDA

Scott Family Members

Robert Walter Scott, Sr. (1861–1929) and Elizabeth Jesse Hughes (1865–1914)
Robert W. Scott, Sr. served five terms in the N.C. General Assembly, and one term in the N.C. State
Senate, starting a legacy of public service. They had 14 children. The following children, and their children, had some bearing on the Family Nurse Practitioner Program at UNC-CH.

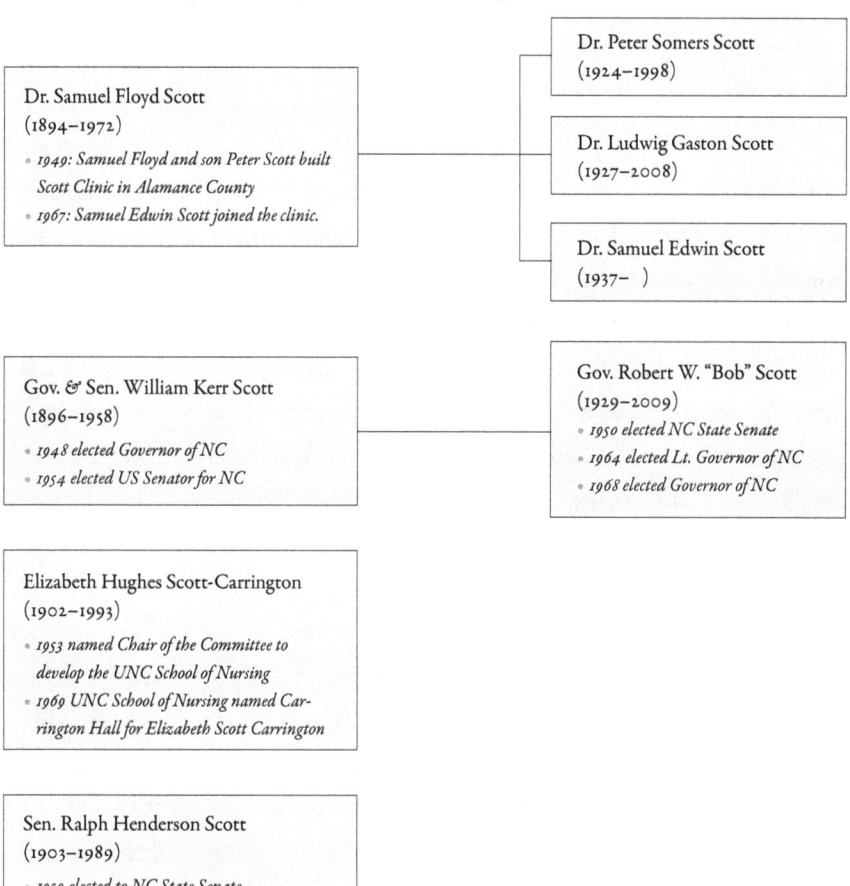

Dr. Samuel Floyd Scott
(1894–1972)
- *1949: Samuel Floyd and son Peter Scott built Scott Clinic in Alamance County*
- *1967: Samuel Edwin Scott joined the clinic.*

Dr. Peter Somers Scott
(1924–1998)

Dr. Ludwig Gaston Scott
(1927–2008)

Dr. Samuel Edwin Scott
(1937–)

Gov. & Sen. William Kerr Scott
(1896–1958)
- *1948 elected Governor of NC*
- *1954 elected US Senator for NC*

Gov. Robert W. "Bob" Scott
(1929–2009)
- *1950 elected NC State Senate*
- *1964 elected Lt. Governor of NC*
- *1968 elected Governor of NC*

Elizabeth Hughes Scott-Carrington
(1902–1993)
- *1953 named Chair of the Committee to develop the UNC School of Nursing*
- *1969 UNC School of Nursing named Carrington Hall for Elizabeth Scott Carrington*

Sen. Ralph Henderson Scott
(1903–1989)
- *1950 elected to NC State Senate*
- *1963 becomes President Pro Tem*

Reference Source: "The Scott Family Collection: Family Tree," accessed January 29, 2020, www.scottcollection.org.

Lead Allies toward a New Order of Things

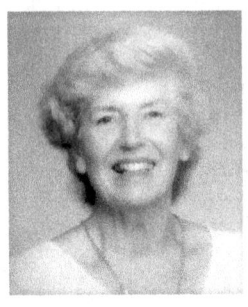 **Mrs. Geneva Warren** (1922–92) was the epitome of the image of the soft-spoken southern woman, modest and reserved, and yet at the same time, she was a powerful political ally and a quick observer of the ways of political influence. She melded the values and customs of the democratic South with her gracious ways and a disciplined determination to achieve health care for her rural community. Her intuitive insights belied her political strategizing; she underplayed her power and influence with an understated modesty. In the end, she became a politician, appointed to several key positions.

Geneva Elizabeth Williams was born in Cumberland County, North Carolina, where her father was a high school principal. As she said, "At that time, like the Methodist preachers, you moved around from time to time."[25] Consequently, in her youth she came to know different parts of North Carolina. At age seventeen, she felt fortunate, given the Depression, to be admitted to the Women's College of the University of North Carolina.[26] She decided, before she finished her study for a degree in education, that she would take the first job she was offered. Then, she thought, after a couple of years at that first job, she would think further about where she really wanted to settle. She took that first offer as a home economics teacher in Prospect Hill.

At age nineteen, she bought a '38 Ford two days before heading off to her new job, stopping first in a nearby town on the way to get her driver's license—all quite gutsy for a woman in that era, a preview of the courage she exhibited throughout her life. Upon arriving at Prospect Hill, North Carolina, she met Joseph Warren—unknown to her but obvious to him at the time, he would be the man she would marry. They did marry and had four children. Joseph Warren was a farmer, merchant, and politician, serving several terms in the state legislature before his untimely death in 1966. Political events had been the fabric of daily life as she and Joseph befriended many politicians. However, she did not consider herself a political person of any sort, but after her husband's death, that changed.

As for as her political involvement, Mrs. Warren reflected, "Although I had been interested and enjoyed it *with* him, to take any part at all myself was completely foreign to me."[27] She decided, though, that she would continue Joseph's work locally by raising funds for the Warren Memorial Clinic in Prospect Hill. Years later, after many conversations with political allies and leaders of UNC, her persistent efforts led to the creation of the Prospect Hill Community Health Center.

Mrs. Warren also decided that she needed to demonstrate for her children the legacy left by her deceased husband. In some way, she had to get involved politically as she vowed not to deprive her children of the rich political heritage so valued by the family. So, Mrs. Warren started attending precinct meetings—with the children in tow. She did not miss a state convention. On election days she took her children by the hand to hotel campaign headquarters. She kept moving in political circles. She would just be there and be seen; she didn't speak. Much to her surprise, she ended up not only as a political activist for the Prospect Hill clinic, but she also served with several well-known politicians in the late '60s and '70s.

"Loyalty" is the key word that best describes politics for Mrs. Warren. Her husband's Democratic Party affiliation and her loyalty to his old friends, the Scotts of neighboring Alamance County, eventually led to her first involvement in a political campaign. She was Caswell County chair for Richardson Pryer's first bid for Congress in 1968. She was the first woman chair of a Democratic congressional district organization in the state; then a member of the State Democratic Party Executive Committee; and finally cocampaign manager of Jim Hunt's race for lieutenant governor. When he was elected governor in 1977, Mrs. Warren consented to serve as Mrs. Hunt's administrative assistant responsible for managing the governor's mansion and social functions.

Mrs. Warren was constantly surprised at her involvement in party politics engendered by her pursuit for her children of the heritage their father had given them. "I would go to a lot of different meetings, be there, and not say anything. That is a secret that people do not know and I found it out in an odd way. You don't have to say a thing to become politically involved. Just be there! Politicians have an eye that skims over a crowd. If they see you at this meeting here, and then in Wilmington, and then in Winston-Salem, they say 'What is it with this woman?' The first thing you know, you're involved."[28]

Geneva Warren is the quintessential gracious southern woman. Despite her achievements, she is unassuming in her description of herself and her accomplishments. She began her political involvement warily, but gradually developed confidence in her diverse political roles. She worked with discipline and persistence to be politically effective, and in the process, she became wise about the nature of politics. She was a powerful political ally in achieving health care for her crossroads community, Prospect Hill. Most of all, she was a most elegant political activist.

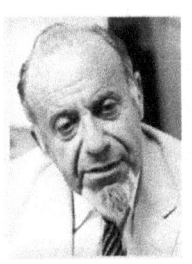

Cecil G. Sheps, MD, MPH (1913–2004), was born in Winnipeg, where he received his MD degree from the University of Manitoba in 1936. After obtaining his Master of Public Health degree at Yale University in 1947, he stayed and worked in the United States throughout the remainder of his career. His first position was as a public health faculty member at the University of North Carolina, 1947 to 1953. He then held significant positions at Beth Israel Hospitals of Boston and New York, Harvard University, University of Pittsburgh, and Mount Sinai School of Medicine in New York.

Sheps returned to UNC again in 1968, this time to direct the new Health Services Research Center (HSRC). Three years later, he became the vice chancellor for health affairs during the formative period of the Nurse Practitioner Program in North Carolina, from 1971 to 1976. Known as one of the founders of the field of health services research, UNC's HSRC was renamed in 1991 as the Cecil G. Sheps Center for Health Services Research.[29]

Dr. Sheps presented a commanding appearance contributed to by his self-assuredness and distinguishing Vandyke beard. His interactive style of influence, however, was informal and conveyed a sense of colleague-ship to all. According to those who worked with him, when he talked with others, they were stimulated—intellectually and even emotion-ally—by what he had to say. It wasn't as much the content of what he said as the conviction with which he said it; he was telling them what he stood for. They realized that all his experience, passion, and commitment were authentic.[30]

Throughout his career, Sheps was dedicated to the public's health, through medical and health service programs. It was his signature goal. And so, Dr. Cecil Sheps influenced reluctant physicians to support newly minted nurse practitioners, and ultimately, he lent his influence to the development of the North Carolina Rural Health Program and the growth of the nurse practitioner movement in the state.

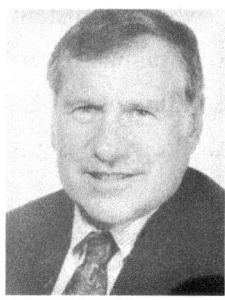

James D. Bernstein (1942–2005). It is near impos-sible to write a brief description of a man who was so well loved and well respected as James (Jim) Ber-nstein. The *North Carolina Medical Journal* dedi-cated twenty-three pages to his life and career, and an entire issue to rural health care—that for which Bernstein is most well-known.[31] But most of what has been written about Bernstein does not reflect his support of and involvement with the UNC Family Nurse Practitioner Program.

President Kennedy's call for Peace Corps volunteers lured Jim Bernstein, just out of college, to Tanza, Morocco—where he not only taught English and physical education for boys, but also where he met and married his wife, Susan, his supportive life-long partner in all his endeavors. Following his Peace Corps tour, a master's degree in hospital administration from the University of Michigan and an internship at Mt. Sinai Hospital in Cleveland preceded his several years in the Indian Health Service.

His assignment, the Santa Fe Service Unit, had responsibility for health and human services in a hospital and outlying health centers for twelve thousand persons in thirteen tribes in New Mexico and Colorado. It was in Santa Fe, working with Dr. Robert Oseasohn, where Bernstein's interest in rural health care began, and where he learned about nurse practitioners. He served on a planning committee for an Oseasohn experiment in which a nurse was trained to deliver primary care for a small town, Estancia, New Mexico. Bernstein was "revved" by these experiences, the foundation for his next steps.

As a Global Community Health Fellow, Jim selected North Carolina as his site for study because of the state's inadequate rural health care as well as its potential resources to change, including the Nurse Practitioner Program that would start coincident with his arrival at UNC in 1970. Bernstein worked with Dr. Cecil Sheps in developing one of the prototype rural nurse practitioner clinics, in Walstonburg, where Bernstein formulated many of his ideas about developing effective rural health services across the state. When the 1973 legislature, at the urging of Governor James Holshouser, Jr., established the Rural Health Program, Bernstein was appointed director.

Within two years after his arrival at UNC, Bernstein became a member of the Family Nurse Practitioner Policy Board—serving on that board for almost a decade. The FNP Program guaranteed student placements for the rural clinics Bernstein and his staff were developing. Bernstein also played a vital role in the closely knit network that shepherded successful nurse practitioner practices across the state. Both programs, the Rural Health Program and the UNC FNP Program, shared reciprocal interests.

Most notable was Bernstein the man. Those who worked with Bernstein knew that excellence was his standard; he would help meet those standards but would not accept anything less. Bernstein was welcoming with whomever he met. Those who knew him well knew without a doubt that he cared about them. His broad, warm smile was embracing.

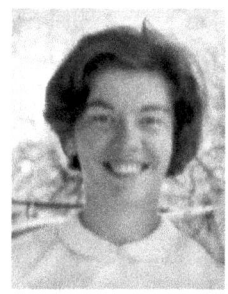

A liberal arts education in the '60s interspersed with preparation as a nurse at Hartford Hospital School of Nursing in Connecticut prepared **Linda Ocker Mashburn** for her leadership in bringing about a health care system for Appalachian Mountain communities in Madison County, North Carolina. She spent her early childhood in the St. Louis and Chicago areas. She attended Mount Holyoke College for three years before beginning nursing studies and completed both her nursing diploma and BA degree in 1965, graduating Phi Beta Kappa with a major in philosophy from Mount Holyoke. She worked summers in Ghana, Nigeria, as a team member with Crossroads Africa and another with the California Migrant Ministry. After two years as head nurse and teacher of nursing students in a hospital in India, she completed an MA in sociology and religion at Columbia University and Union Theological Seminary. And then she found her real mission.

Linda Mashburn coordinated forty health fairs in as many Appalachian counties in five states while she was mobile health fair coordinator for the United Presbyterian Church and Council of the Southern Appalachian Mountains in Berea, Kentucky. During the four winters between the various fairs, she assisted communities with developing permanent health care solutions and coordinated activities of the council's Health Commission. She became familiar with the health care model of the Frontier Nursing Service in Clay and Perry counties, Kentucky, and describes her zealous wish to implement such a model.

Hot Springs, North Carolina, one of the health fair sites, seemed to be ready for a clinic. Their timing matched Linda's readiness to settle in one place after 160,000 miles of Volkswagen travel and living in a tiny travel trailer for four years in Berea. She became project director of the Hot Springs Health Program in 1971 and by 1972 developed three clinics offering a range of services to include medical and dental out-patient care, home health care, health education, and transportation. She continued as advisor and board member to the Hot Springs, Walnut, and Laurel clinics, and helped the board expand services to the Marshall area.

Her enthusiastic commitment, persistence, and dedication to the health of Appalachian communities, and most especially to residents of Madison County, North Carolina, was contagious—which is why so many others joined her cause. She exemplified the best of public health nursing standards; her care and concern were for every individual as well as all for those of the community. Her natural inclinations and public health nursing background were later complemented by completion of a Master of Public Health degree—the latter while she was directing and serving on the board of the Hot Springs Health Program she had developed.

CHAPTER FIVE

The University Primes: Bringing Vision to Life

Throughout the 1960s, several leaders at the University of North Carolina at Chapel Hill (UNC) Schools of Nursing, Medicine, and Public Health advocated for the nurse practitioner concept. Lucy Conant had a vision. Glenn Pickard had a vision. Cecil Sheps had a vision. Julia Watkins[1] had a vision. All had visions, each with some variation on the same theme. The leaders in these schools had to merge their visions and their ideas by planning and giving structure to an actual family nurse practitioner program. And they also had to find a way to organize a system to get a clinic in Prospect Hill up and running. Designing curriculum for educational programs was something they did almost daily. Planning, opening, and managing a clinic was another matter, however. Increasing support within the university, securing outside start-up funding, and turning a few hurdles into opportunities provided the requisite impetus to develop the Family Nurse Practitioner (FNP) Program into a working reality.

THE DIVISION OF HEALTH SCIENCES

In the 1960s, the University of North Carolina at Chapel Hill articulated its responsibility to help solve the state's health problems. This pledge was not mere rhetoric, for the new Division of Health Sciences championed this commitment. The university's Health Sciences Division came about because of concern over the poor health status of the state's three and a half million citizens as revealed through the large numbers of World War II draftees who failed the health and fitness criteria to serve. When the legislature created the Health Sciences Division, it gave the division a mandate to serve the citizens of the state and provide improved health care to the state's citizens by training more physicians, nurses, and other health care providers. All the health science schools—nursing, medicine, dentistry, pharmacy, and public health—in varying ways endorsed this mandate from the state.

At the same time, communities organized to search for solutions to their own health care problems. Ultimately, however, new clinic buildings and physician recruitment campaigns failed, so community leaders approached the nearest academic health center for help. When several North Carolina communities approached the university asking for help in finding a doctor, their pleas did not fall on deaf ears.

Fortunately, the Division of Health Affairs' new and energetic leaders in the Schools of Medicine, Nursing, and Public Health created a climate for innovative approaches to solving the state's health care system problems. They, in turn, helped communities think differently about solutions. Fortunately, community leaders also found committed faculty in the university swimming against the tide of traditional, more mainstream academic approaches to solving community problems, and so community leaders found hope and saw new possibilities. These nontraditional faculty, and their community counterparts, became leaders and supporters of the nurse practitioner movement.

THE MEDICAL SCHOOL

In 1952, progressive faculty with new ideas about preventive, continuing care, and primary care medicine were recruited by Dean Berryhill. This new breed of young physicians organized some hospital clinics along "general" clinic lines, not wanting to follow the specialty clinic route.

This swim upstream led to the continuing care clinic demonstration project, where it became accepted practice to have nurses and social workers increasingly involved in patient care activities.

Glenn Pickard joined the continuing care project when he returned to UNC in 1965. He began giving nurses extensive informal instruction in physical assessment; in turn, the nurses took on increasing responsibility for the monitoring and care of chronically ill patients in the continuing care clinic. Over time nurses became the primary caretakers for patients, both within the clinic and in their homes. In addition to general satisfaction with patient outcomes among patients, physicians, nurses, and social workers, the project also resulted in very positive physician–nurse interaction and collaboration. As we now know, the expanded role of the nurse in that continuing care project turned out to be the precursor to the nurse practitioner role.

Despite the success of the continuing care project, expansion of this project and its goals—comprehensive primary care to local residents and development of an advanced nursing role—were inhibited by counter forces within the Medical Center. Even though more and more people were coming to the hospital clinics with common primary care problems—respiratory infections, diabetes, hypertension, etc.—the more specialty-oriented physicians thought these types of patients unduly overloaded the clinics. The increasing numbers of medical students and residents needing specialty patient care experiences took priority, in the view of the specialist physicians, and therefore the specialty-oriented clinics could not accommodate those patients needing primary care services.

Yet some recognized the growing need for primary care. Pickard said we realized that "we could never delegate to the nurse a consistent level of [greater] responsibility. We would never find out what a nurse practitioner could do if she kept her practice within the limiting parameters of the institution."[2] Although the continuing care project was successful, particularly as a prelude to establishing the nurse practitioner role and effective nurse–physician collaboration, the university Medical Center was not going to be the best place for continuing experimentation with primary care delivery systems and expanded nursing roles. The majority of medical faculty did not view primary care or advancing nurses' clinical roles as priorities. Those opposed felt it was not in keeping with their view of the university Medical Center as a highly specialized medical referral center. But fortunately, there was support at higher levels within the medical school.

Dean Berryhill's successor in 1964, Dr. Isaac Taylor, was also supportive of the direction the cadre of community-oriented faculty were taking in expanding the role of nurses. Dr. Louis Welt, internationally renowned for his renal transport research, was now chair of the Department of Medicine, and thus he was a dominant figure in the medical school and influential among his colleagues. He fostered collaboration between medicine and nursing and supported the development of the nurse practitioner. Welt knew that physicians would be trained as specialists and not as primary care providers, and therefore, they would not be prepared to practice in rural community clinics. To Welt, the nurse practitioner seemed a more reasonable answer to communities exerting pressure on the medical school for more caregivers. Important as his support was, however, it was not the degree of backing needed to move toward a formal program to prepare nurse practitioners.

Dr. Glenn Pickard, while chief resident in medicine, and later Dr. Larry (Lawrence) Cutchin, succeeding Pickard as chief resident in medicine, went to Lou Welt to get his blessing about developing training and a defined role for nurses in primary care. His endorsement was critical, but this did not come overnight. Even so, Pickard was not discouraged. "During the time I was chief resident and first on the faculty, I had a whole series of documents about planning for primary care in the local area, and I would send these missives off to Dr. Welt and Bill [William] Cromartie, associate dean, School of Medicine, and Ike [Taylor], and they just kind of thumbed their noses at them. We just kept hammering and hammering and hammering."[3] Meanwhile, Pickard and Bryan persisted, maintaining their support for the continuing care clinic.

Ultimately, Pickard and others realized that primary care had to be offered "out there"—in local community clinics and not at the university Medical Center clinics. Further, they also understood that a formalized NP training program was needed if both the NP idea and rural clinics were going to materialize. But until a formal FNP program was established, Pickard kept meeting with Geneva Warren, promising what he hoped he could deliver, and hoping that Geneva Warren could deliver political support and funding from legislators in Raleigh.

THE SCHOOL OF PUBLIC HEALTH

The School of Public Health supported the FNP Program from its early beginnings. In fact, during the first eight years of the program, the FNP Program took pride in billing itself as the "Family Nurse Practitioner Program of the University of North Carolina at Chapel Hill, School of Nursing, School of Medicine, and School of Public Health." Support from the School of Public Health was particularly important during the years 1968–72, and its sponsorship was ongoing until September 1978 when the School of Nursing moved the FNP Program into its mainstream degree-granting offerings.

Early support came naturally. Several of the community-oriented medical faculty who had been recruited by Dean Berryhill held joint appointments in the School of Public Health (SPH).[4] Here their interests converged with those of the nonphysician public health faculty who supported the development of community-based primary care services and training of nurse practitioners. Many of these medical–public health faculty were involved in the continuing care demonstration project at the hospital clinics. They shared their experiences and advocacy for a different model of care with their public health colleagues during informal discussions, weekly lunch research conferences, and collaboration on research projects.

UNC's School of Public Health was one of the top public health schools in the country, and it had its share of influential faculty with clout nationally. Margaret Dolan, director of the Department of Public Health Nursing in the School of Public Health, was one such person—a strong supporter of the nurse practitioner, and a powerful one at that. She saw the nurse practitioner as a natural extension of the public health nurse. Dolan was politically active, serving as president of the American Nurses Association in 1962 through 1964. Later, in 1973, she became president of the American Public Health Association, an unusual post for a woman and even more so for a nurse.

In the late '60s, Dolan organized a series of informal get-togethers of public health nursing leaders from around the country. According to Carolyn Williams,

> the initial participants included Dolan, as organizer; Dr. Doris Roberts, then director of the Nursing Practice Branch of the Division of Nursing; Lee [Loretta] Ford, who at that time was chair of the Department of Public Health Nursing at the University of Colorado; Lillian Ostrand, chair of the Department of Public Health Nursing at the University of Michigan School of Public Health; the chair of the Department of the University of Minnesota School of Public Health, Barbara Leonard, who recently retired about two years ago; Virginia Ohlson, who chaired the Department of Public Health Nursing at the University of Illinois; and myself. We called ourselves the "Mini-Forum," and the

first meeting, sometime in 1968, was in Margaret Dolan's living room, and continued for several years, often in tandem with other national conferences. Their discussions focused on public health nursing issues and the new nurse practitioner role.[5]

These national discussions served to strengthen Dolan's conviction that the nurse practitioner was a viable and effective provider of primary care. She recognized the health care problems in North Carolina. She saw public health nurses as a key to the solution and thought that nurse practitioner skills would be useful additions to their preparation. The group's effort focused on alleviating problems of inadequate quantity and quality of primary care. In Dolan's view, expanded training of public health nurses as nurse practitioners was a prominent and necessary part of solving the country's primary care crisis.[6]

At home, Dolan encouraged her faculty as well as nurses in other departments in the School of Public Health to become involved with the evolving program. As noted in chapter 1, four of them (Aabel, Efird, Hood, and Wilkman) were admitted to the pilot class of the FNP Program, and public health nurses continued to enroll in the program in future years. Jessie Pergrin, a nurse, enrolled in the SPH epidemiology doctoral program, and got involved in various ways with the School of Nursing and later with the development of the Walstonburg community clinic. All of the SPH faculty and some of the students began to discuss needed curricular requirements for a training program. It is difficult to trace all the ways the faculty and nurses-as-students got involved, but they were ardently involved in advocacy.

Perhaps the most significant School of Public Health endorsement came from two faculty, Julia Watkins and Marie McIntyre. They were first to respond to requests from Robert Huntley and Frank Williams[7] for nurses to work in the continuing care demonstration project. They each became one of the nursing codirectors of the FNP Program, Watkins serving the longest, succeeding McIntyre. In those positions, they held faculty appointments in the School of Nursing, as well as in the School of Public Health.

Except for McIntyre and Watkins, who were intimately involved with curricular development and the training program, other public health faculty contributed to the Nurse Practitioner Program's development by conducting research and documenting the need for primary care services. And the support from Greenberg and Dolan should not be understated either. Dr. Bernard Greenberg was appointed dean of the SPH in 1972; from that year forward, his support was unwavering. And the impact of a public endorsement by a renowned figure in public health and nursing, both locally and nationally, namely Dolan, was incalculable. These men and women were not on the front line of teaching and practice, but the support of such widely recognized and highly respected professionals was of significant consequence.

THE NURSING SCHOOL

Support for anything close to the nurse practitioner idea in the nursing school before Lucy Conant's appointment as dean in 1968 was almost nonexistent—except for that of a few willing to buck the tide. Most of the faculty were committed to ongoing responsibilities in the undergraduate and master's programs and endorsed the traditional goals of these programs. A few of the tide-bucking faculty joined their like-minded physicians in the continuing care clinic, namely Betty West and Faye Pickard, as well as Marie McIntyre from the SPH. Faye and Marie decided to spend time each week in the continuing care clinic, developing their clinical practice by working with Drs. Glenn Pickard and Jim Bryan. Faye said the physicians used her to see what nurses could already do and what else they needed to learn to practice in an expanded role.

We were all surprised that with just a little information on lung sounds, how many more decisions I could make about patient care than I had been able to make previously. One patient I remember making a home visit to fairly soon after his discharge from the hospital. After listening to what was happening to him and listening to his lung sounds and so forth, I called Glenn [Pickard], who got hold of the admitting resident, and we arranged to have the patient admitted. Several days later, in Grand Rounds, the note that I had written on the patient's chart was read by Tom Barnett [attending physician]. He then commented that this note—no one imagined it might be [mine]—shows what a good public health nurse can do.[8]

Most of the nursing faculty, though, were not supportive of the continuing care clinic and increasing responsibilities for nurses because they had not heard of this project. Betty West, though, had because she held dual appointments with the School of Nursing and as a public health nurse with the Chatham County Health Department. In the latter capacity, she often communicated with Bryan or Pickard about her patients. When she heard of their continuing care clinic "experiment," she was eager to jump on board. Faye Pickard, of course, heard about the clinic from her husband, Glenn. She noted that most often, she and Glenn would discuss their ideas, agreements, and disagreements at home. Their eldest daughter recalled many a discussion around the dinner table about nurse practitioners improving the health care system.[9] Faye Pickard was most supportive of expanding nurses' responsibilities, and she wanted to establish a practice in the continuing care clinic so that she could provide new experiences for nursing graduate students.

Several other School of Nursing (SON) faculty supported the nurse practitioner concept and worked together with faculty from the SOM and SPH to propose curricular content for the new program. Linda

Staurovsky, a master's-prepared certified midwife recently appointed to the SON faculty, eagerly joined in this work. As a midwife, she easily understood the potential of nurse practitioners providing primary care. Carol Fray, an expert in pathophysiology and a new faculty member from Cornell University, also joined the curricular planning group. Fray was an important and specifically targeted recruit by Dean Conant.

When Dean Conant arrived at UNC in 1968, she took quick note that there were no faculty of color in the School of Nursing, and just as quickly, she was determined to change that. She asked current faulty whether they knew of or had contacts with nursing faculty of color who were teaching at other schools. One faculty member, Amie Modigh, recommended Fray highly, and after visits to North Carolina and interviews with existing faculty, Fray was offered a faculty appointment in the School of Nursing.[10] Four months later, in January 1969, Conant welcomed Fray, the first black faculty member, to the School of Nursing.[11] Fray joined Pickard (Faye) and Staurovsky on the interdisciplinary curriculum planning committee.

Except for these few, the views of most nursing faculty reflected the dominant viewpoint of organized nursing—which did not support the nurse practitioner concept at that time. In the mid-sixties, there was debate over the use of the terms "expanded" vs. "extended" nursing roles. Some interpreted "expanded" as expansion into the territory of medical practice; others interpreted "extended" as an extension of the physician's arm, and thus, as an assistant to the physician. The introduction of the "physician assistant" titling by Duke University in 1967 muddied the water even more. Was this new role intended to be an advanced nursing role, or was it to be another step toward assisting doctors with their work? Reaction to the nurse practitioner concept among nurses across the country ranged from fierce opposition to serious skepticism, and only sometimes, a tentative approval. There was at that time little whole-hearted support.

In reality, though, these debates served to camouflage some of the reasons underlying the resistance to the nurse practitioner concept within organized nursing. Nurses in the fifties struggled and fought to gain independence from medicine; they viewed the nurse practitioner idea as a threat to those gains. Moving nursing education from hospital-based and physician-controlled diploma programs to colleges and universities, as independent schools of nursing, was just gaining ground. This was certainly true for the School of Nursing at UNC. The original proposal for a new School of Nursing put the nursing program within the School of Medicine, under the dean of the medical school. Elizabeth Scott Carrington, of the influential Scott family referenced in chapter 3, learned of this proposal and garnered the support of a few influential business and political leaders to call for an independent School of Nursing. With a baccalaureate degree and Master of Science in Nursing degree from the University of Pennsylvania, Carrington knew that a superior program would only come from an independent School of Nursing—and she lobbied fiercely for that. As Mr. William Friday, the president of the University of North Carolina system for thirty years, famously said on many occasions, "Once Elizabeth Carrington makes up her mind about something and takes it on as a mission, you had best agree and step aside."

Nursing professionals had had to fight to control their own educational programs; thus, they did not want to lose ground. Further, nurses sought recognition as independent professionals, meaning that their work was not solely or entirely dependent on physicians or their orders. However, the nurse practitioner idea drew opposition from other nurses who feared a return to physician domination of nursing education because, initially, much of the teaching in the new nurse practitioner programs had to be done by physicians. Adding fuel to the fire, the close relationship between nurses and physicians in the new nurse practitioner programs clouded the drive by others seeking recognition as independent

professionals. Many of the voices of opposition came from nursing educators, however, and not from practicing nurses.

Years before the nurse practitioner movement, nurses and physicians
who worked closely together clinically saw themselves as a team. Many
of these nurse–doctor pairs, without fanfare, recognition, or legal sanction, had already drifted in the direction of expanded nursing roles. The
arrival of coronary care units (CCUs) in the early 1960s, quietly and of
necessity, authenticated expanded nursing roles. To save lives with new
CCU monitoring technologies, treatment had to be used immediately,
and nurses were the professionals who were present 24/7 to provide these
treatments. So, CCU nurses were trained to rapidly diagnose and treat
life-threatening arrhythmias—a major shift in the usual responsibilities
of nurses.[12] Fifty years later, celebrating the advent of CCUs, Fye confirmed this major shift in nursing practice boundaries, referring to it as
nurse empowerment. He further noted that "The advent and diffusion of
the CCU would transform the care of patients, the careers of cardiologists, and the boundaries of nursing practice in less than a decade."[13]

The boundaries of nursing practice have never been static or cast in
stone. But in the years immediately preceding the beginning of the nurse
practitioner movement, the boundaries of coronary care nurses stretched
far and wide and affected the boundaries and relationships of both nurses
and physicians. Coronary care nurses and cardiologists alike fostered this
development without raising the ire of the professional associations or
the nursing education establishment.

A few years later in the mid-sixties, shortly after the rise of CCUs,
and into the early seventies, the nurse practitioner movement tested the
professional associations' tolerance for further expanding the boundaries of nursing practice. The official voices of organized medicine and
nursing did not include those practicing nurses who were stretching and
testing new boundaries in CCUs, but the official proclamations were

so expansive that nurse practitioner proponents as well as their nursing opponents were outraged.

American Medical Association (AMA) proclamations were often the most inflammatory to nurses. The exclamation in *Look Magazine* in September 1966, and seconded by the American Medical Association, that a new type of practitioner was "more than a nurse, less than a doctor,"[14] infuriated virtually all nurses. That was not their only *faux pas*. Suggesting that nurses in expanded roles could resolve the doctor crisis in America certainly added fuel to the fire. Of course, the American Nurses Association had to fight back.[15] Within this rising storm of discontent nurse practitioner advocates had to tread their way very carefully.

The groundwork for nurse practitioners had been laid in the UNC Medical Center continuing care project. And now a group of physicians was exerting pressure on the School of Nursing for a new training program. In addition, Prospect Hill was waiting impatiently for nurse practitioners to open their clinic. However, focused planning and negotiation for a nurse practitioner program did not begin until Dr. Lucy Conant became dean of the nursing school in 1968.

Conant had practiced public health nursing in both the United States and England and had taught community health at Yale University. Her interests in expanding nursing's role in the community matched those evolving in the School of Public Health and the School of Medicine, and the select few in the nursing school. In addition to her interest in the nurse practitioner concept, her appointment as dean carried with it the explicit charge of strengthening the school's association with the other health science schools. Strengthening these relationships was a stated and essential ingredient to a nurse practitioner program.

But Conant did not find unanimous endorsement of the nurse practitioner concept from the nursing faculty, which mirrored those of many other nurse educators and leaders in the country. She had several discussions with Glenn Pickard after she arrived, which raised Conant's awareness of the urgency for a formal program to prepare nurse practitioners. While Conant worked to establish a meaningful formal relationship with the dean of the medical school, she encouraged the faculty involved in the continuing care project to continue their informal ties with the medical faculty.

As the medical and nursing faculty continued to work together, Dean Conant held many discussions with Dean Isaac Taylor to strengthen established relationships between the nursing and medical schools. In 1969, Deans Conant and Taylor formalized a commitment to developing a nurse practitioner training program by appointing an ad hoc curriculum committee, composed of both medical and nursing faculty. Their charge to faculty was the first official statement that there would be a family nurse practitioner training program.

Committee members were those faculty who had experimented with interdisciplinary collaboration and expanded nursing roles in the continuing care project. Members from the medical school included Glenn Pickard, Jim Bryan, Robert Shaw, Robert Smith, and Larry Cutchin—a resident. Cutchin would soon become a proponent of the nurse practitioner concept in eastern North Carolina. Nursing school representation included Faye Pickard, Carol Fray, and Linda Staurowsky, a certified nurse-midwife. The School of Public Health's involvement was formalized by the joint appointments of two public health nurse faculty, Marie McIntyre and Judy Watkins, to the School of Nursing. They, as well as Margaret Dolan, were appointed to the ad hoc committee.

The ad hoc curriculum committee discussed the nurse practitioner concept and curricular issues. They focused on what *additional* knowledge nurse practitioner students would need. After all, as registered nurses they were not starting with a blank slate. They identified the requisite assessment and diagnostic knowledge required based on their experiences in the continuing care clinic. To complete this task, various curriculum subgroups spun off the main committee. They needed input for pediatric content. And there was a nursing curriculum subgroup, addressing the question: Is there a need for *additional* nursing content, and if so, what?

Soon, however, the continuous need for interpretation of the nurse practitioner role made a definition of the term "nurse practitioner" essential. How could they plan a curriculum without knowing what a nurse practitioner was? Further, as word got around about the nature of this "nurse practitioner" endeavor, no one could respond knowledgeably and consistently without an agreed-upon definition. Intensifying the immediate need for those working on the nurse practitioner curriculum committee at UNC was the rapid development of physician assistant programs at Duke University and in other places in the country. Further, the general use of the term "physician extender" to describe both nurse practitioners and physician assistants compounded the confusion in distinguishing between their practice roles. A definition of the intended product, the family nurse practitioner, was imperative.

Consequently, the ad hoc curriculum committee diverted their focus to formulating a definition. This committee, from its very beginning, functioned as a consensus-gathering committee. But now their task was quite different. The committee struggled with describing the problem, explaining the need, and defining the nurse practitioner role. Nonetheless, within the committee, equality between disciplines, mutual respect, and compromise was established as the basis for achieving common goals. Agreement on a definition was a critical test of the interdisciplinary collaboration foundational to offering a nurse practitioner program—and to nurse practitioner practice itself.

Members of the ad hoc curriculum committee were consistent in their understanding of nurse practitioners and what their role ought to be. There was consensus on preparing a generalist who could provide care to patients of all ages. However, putting their ideas on paper was another matter. An early draft referred to the nurse practitioner's role as an "independent" one. This word was appealing to nursing faculty; the medical faculty committee members did not oppose it, but they were concerned about having to defend it both to their colleagues in the medical school and to the medical establishment outside the university. And the support of the medical establishment would be crucial for laying the foundation for a successful nurse practitioner movement.

Another compromise was also needed; nursing committee members opposed the word "supervision." They believed it implied the supervision of nursing practice by physicians. The nursing faculty knew such a definition would be death to the nurse practitioner idea within the nursing community. There had to be support within both the medical and nursing establishments. After much thoughtful discussion, in November 1969, a compromise was achieved, the first of many between medicine and nursing that had to be made to move the program forward. The compromise phrasing was "in collaboration with designated physicians who supervise their medical activities." Thus, "supervision" was limited to the medical aspects of the nurse practitioner role, and "collaboration" pointed to a new relationship between nurses and physicians. The red flags of "independence" and "supervision" were averted. The ad hoc committee adopted a definition of what they wanted the product (i.e., the nurse practitioner) to be:

Family Nurse Practitioners are registered nurses who have completed a formal program of study which qualifies them to function with a combination of traditional nursing skills, such as counseling and teaching, and newly acquired medical skills, such as diagnosis and treatment. They are prepared to provide health care to patients of all ages, chiefly in ambulatory settings, in collaboration with designated physicians who supervise their medical activities within established protocols of care.

The practice of Family Nurse Practitioners is oriented to the needs and concerns of consumers and includes preventive health maintenance as well as medical management. They use knowledge of the complex interplay of health, social, and economic factors to make personal interventions on behalf of patients and families and to use appropriate community agencies. Their concerns extend to the identification of the health needs of the entire community, and they contribute to the development of needed resources and programs.[16]

Margaret Dolan could not attend the ad hoc committee meeting when the definition was on the agenda. She asked Judy Watkins to attend in her stead. Judy went to the meeting "expecting fireworks." She continued, "I remember it started out with 'A nurse practitioner is an independent practitioner,' and I really thought the fireworks would hit.... [T]here weren't fireworks, but that one sentence was changed to read 'independent functions.'"[17] The ad hoc committee passed the test of interdisciplinary collaboration!

The developing Nurse Practitioner Program was given a high degree of administrative protection in the School of Nursing and kept out of mainstream discussions to hasten its implementation. Dean Conant, Faye Pickard, and others shared the belief from the beginning that the Nurse Practitioner Program should eventually be offered as part of a graduate degree program to produce more broadly prepared clinicians and administrators. However, the immediate needs of underserved communities took priority. Therefore, the new program started as a continuing education offering to save it from attack and tampering by opponents. The general faculty of the school did not hold approval authority over continuing education programs.

Most of the early nurse practitioner programs began as continuing education "certificate" programs where they enjoyed safe harbor
from faculty opposition. Such administrative protection contributed
to the divisiveness within the nursing profession over the legitimacy of
this new nursing role. Opponents criticized the programs because the
scope, depth, and prerequisite credentialing would not be scrutinized
by the usual academic degree-granting accreditation mechanisms and
because they were seen as physician dominated. However, it was the
only option for many new nurse practitioner programs. Without the
administrative protection of a continuing education offering, any new
nurse practitioner program would have been jeopardized by a lack of
faculty endorsement.

Because program planning was effectively insulated, key nursing faculty who strongly espoused advanced practice but not the nurse practitioner idea were bypassed in the rush to get the first pilot practitioner curriculum launched. Betty Sue Johnson, who had been strongly influenced
by Thelma Ingles, a member of the Duke nursing faculty who in the 1950s
emphasized advanced clinical preparation and practice, was, ironically, one
of those opposing the program. Before joining the University of North
Carolina nursing faculty, Dr. Johnson had been associated with Ingles in a
project demonstrating a practice–educator nursing role at Duke.

At the University of North Carolina, Johnson was director of the
graduate program in the School of Nursing. She firmly believed in the
necessity for a high level of clinical competency and also in the value of
physician collaboration but saw the Nurse Practitioner Program as physician dominated and thus primarily nonnursing. In Johnson's view, "It got
off on a very bad foot because it politically made itself out to be a 'high-
faluting, nobody can touch us with a ten-foot pole. We're special. We're
new. We're going to change the world. We don't want to have anything
to do with nursing. We're different. We're not nurses. We're going to be

FNPs.'"[18] Johnson's view was shared by many in nursing who supported advanced clinical practice, but not nurse practitioners as it was being defined and developed.

Referring to the total faculty, Johnson recalled, "We never once approved the curriculum. It was never once sent to the executive committee." In Johnson's view, the curricular components were in place in the undergraduate and graduate programs to eventually offer the curriculum in the graduate program. She reflected:

> I think [the curriculum] could have been turned around in three years. I still believe the more independent the practice, the higher the education has to be because you're away from your support system.... What we probably would have done would be to set it up in the master's program and added on another year to clinical practice—I wouldn't have allowed it unless they had a year of internship because of the degree of independence.[19,20]

Faculty also worried that this new curricular sibling might be thriving at some cost to the school's more traditional endeavors, so they didn't like their lack of participation in decision making. The ad hoc curriculum committee did ask for suggestions on content for the nurse practitioner curriculum from each of the nursing school's clinical departments, but it was the interdisciplinary ad hoc committee who decided the appropriateness of the content and who eventually designed the nurse practitioner curriculum. Faculty also feared that the funds necessary for the FNP Program would ultimately dilute funding for the existing undergraduate and graduate programs. As it developed, the Nurse Practitioner Program engendered ample new funding, although the uncertainty and timing of its arrival, with notification of approval for funding coming during the summer months when most faculty were on vacation, contributed to the mystery of the program's source of support. In retrospect, though, the insulation of the program allowed the small, decision-making ad hoc committee to take fast action without time-consuming and broadly representative, albeit democratic, planning.

THE MERGER OF FORCES, FUNDING, AND FACULTY

Much ground had been tilled. Medical faculty were on board and working on curriculum plans. Public health faculty also worked on curricular issues. They also offered endorsement and encouraged students to enroll in the program, and two nursing faculty ultimately became intimately involved with the program. Lucy Conant secured support from her counterpart, the medical school dean, and together they institutionalized an "ad hoc committee" to bring together those wanting to move the Nurse Practitioner Program forward. This later represented a major "official" institutional commitment. Despite all these successes, though, a few hurdles remained. Faculty—primarily nursing faculty. Funding. And endorsement by key university power brokers. However, these hurdles were cleared, almost simultaneously, in early 1970.

Nursing Faculty

Conant had managed to secure agreement that the School of Nursing would be the home for the FNP Program, not the School of Public Health, as Margaret Dolan had championed. A belief among some nurse practitioner supporters was that the new NP role was a legitimization of what public health nurses were already doing, and that a formalized NP program would serve to enable and expand the public health nurse's role. But there was no doubt in Conant's mind; the nurse practitioner role would lead to enhanced role and boundary changes in the practice of all nurses.

I felt *strongly* that it was an expanded clinical role in nursing, not just public health nursing, and that what we might do in the primary care area would affect the development in other clinical nursing areas—pediatrics, nurse-midwifery, geriatrics, etc. All along I saw the FNP as a cooperative program but one that should be based in a School of Nursing, and this was what I fought for.[21]

There was easy consensus that the program be led by two codirectors: one a nurse and the other a physician. Conant did not have many options for the nurse codirector among the School of Nursing faculty. Faye Pickard was an obvious choice. However, as Faye Pickard recalls, she and Conant talked about this and together they decided Pickard could be of more help continuing to work in the graduate program.

Both Lucy and I believed very strongly that the FNP Program needed to be built into the graduate program. We saw my staying involved with the graduate program as one way of doing this.... We felt very strongly that it should be built in as an elective opportunity in the graduate program from the beginning. At that time, I was not only chair of the med–surg department but was also heading the med–surg component of the graduate program.[22]

Conant did not have many other options among School of Nursing faculty. Most early programs faced similar dilemmas. None of their faculty members were prepared as nurse practitioners; in fact, there were very few prepared NPs serving as faculty in the entire country in the late '60s. The few other nursing faculty who might be interested in leading the program were already heavily committed to the ever-expanding baccalaureate and graduate programs. Judy Watkins recalled a meeting in which Conant asked if anyone might be interested.

We were very interested, Marie [McIntrye] and I in particular. I have often thought about the fact that I didn't get a feeling of the School of Nursing [faculty] being that interested. The reason I'm saying this is that we had a meeting of what turned out to be the policy committee—I think it was called that at first, sort of a task force. That must have been in 1969–70,[23] I forget which one. Lucy said we need somebody, a nurse, to work full-time with the program. I don't think she used the word "director." Do you know of anyone who would like to do it? The interesting thing was why would she have said that if she really had had a lot of interest on her faculty? I remember Marie and I both raised our hands and said we'd be interested.[24]

These two School of Public Health faculty members were not just interested. As Watkins said, "Marie McIntyre and I in particular were vitally interested."[25] McIntyre became the first "nurse" program codirector. In actual practice, however, the program simply listed two codirectors: Marie McIntyre, RN, MPH, and Glenn Pickard, MD. One hurdle cleared.

Funding

Funding the program was even more difficult than identifying program faculty. Audrey Booth, a nursing school faculty member, worked for the North Carolina Regional Medical Program (NCRMP) as director for health professions education. She was able to secure funds for the School of Nursing from the NCRMP for curriculum planning, which was needed but certainly not sufficient to start a new program. The B-budget[26] secured in 1969 by the university brought money to the School of Medicine to prepare primary care physicians and included funds for physician support and involvement in the Family Nurse Practitioner Program. But it wasn't enough to fund a training program *and* fund a new clinic. In the first year, those two were tightly linked.

Glenn Pickard was getting nervous. He had promised Geneva Warren that nurse practitioners and doctors would be in Prospect Hill in 1969, and when that could not materialize, he promised 1970. When the 1970 target could not be met, Pickard promised spring 1971. Fortunately, this time, Pickard did not have to extend his promise again. The program began in the fall of 1970, and in the spring of 1971, nurse practitioners and physicians were in Prospect Hill. Pickard and Conant knew they could manage to put together a curriculum to begin teaching FNPs as Booth offered sufficient start-up funds from the NCRMP. But they had no idea how they would fund a clinic. Even so, funding for a clinic did materialize, though not in a way that Pickard, Conant, or anyone else had foreseen.

Paul Alston came and courted the university in much the same way that Geneva Warren had done several years earlier. Paul Alston was the head of the local OEO (Office of Economic Opportunity), one of Lyndon Johnson's Great Society programs. Alston came "on a mission to the dean, like Ms. Geneva, and said, 'Is the university interested in establishing a proper system of primary care for the local populations?'"[27]

OEO programs in other parts of the country were successful in creating economic and social opportunity through the vehicle of health care. The national OEO office felt similar programs were needed in the South. Alston was an astute politician and he saw an opportunity. He developed a relationship with the director of the Orange County Health Department, Dr. Dave Garland—who at that time had jurisdiction over several surrounding counties. According to Pickard, "Paul [Alston] came over, saw the dean, got referred to us, and we smelled money."[28] Pickard continued:

I think, realistically, had we had the funds, we would never have looked at OEO, because OEO at that time had already achieved a record of being anti-intellectual, anti-university, anti-research, anti- most of the things the university stood for. There was an acknowledged difference of agendas between OEO, trying to provide social change through health care, and the university. We had been encouraged very favorably by Lou [Welt] and others, but their whole vision was that if the university does this, it's got to be done in the name of teaching and research.... You've got to have a research interest and an educational interest.... So, we viewed OEO with some disdain, but by the same token we appreciated the fact that there were lots of poor people and we didn't really have the funds to provide care for them at the level we wanted.[29]

Glenn Pickard, Robert Smith, Bob Shaw, and Bob Huntley had a series of meetings with Alston and Garland. They decided they should undertake this project, a partnership, really, in a serious way and truly test the nurse practitioner–rural care model without fiscal constraints. Taylor, the dean, and Welt, the chair of medicine, got a little nervous—as Pickard says, "They got wet feet." Here were Pickard, Smith, Shaw, and Huntley, young and eager and ready to take on the world with their beliefs. Admittedly, "[W]e didn't know a damn thing about running a clinic." Nor did they have any idea about how to organize a community clinic. Taylor and Welt decided to look for somebody who knew something about the economics and organization of health care systems. Enter Glenn Wilson, who was parachuted in as a consultant to help put together a strategy for organizing the OEO-sponsored clinics and utilizing nurse practitioners.

Wilson, previously director of Kaiser in Cleveland, was working as a freelance consultant. He had gotten to know Taylor, Welt, and Sheps; he seemed to them to be the right person to help the university through this process. Pickard described Wilson as "a 'for-real' person, and I think this is why he hit it off with yours truly and some of the other people. We were not the traditional academicians wanting to study about it and not do it. We really wanted to get out there and do it. So, he found a collegial relationship that he appreciated, and we found him to be a boon companion because he actually had organized health care [programs]."[30] Pickard recalled:

We had a famous breakfast meeting with Floyd Denny [chair of pediatrics], Lou Welt [chair of medicine], and Ike Taylor [dean]—they were the power structure of the medical school.... It was mainly Floyd and Lou and Ike, Bill Cromartie [associate dean] ... I forget who else was there. It was one Sunday morning at some ungodly early hour in the old hospital cafeteria where Glenn [Wilson] put on a hallucinated organizational structure for how Orange–Chatham—the new name for the OEO-sponsored clinics—would be created and run, as a vehicle. Lou Welt had at that point written several scathing editorial-like pieces.... They'd certainly gone around the hospital interoffice memorandum route. It had become the acknowledged policy of the institution that the only service the university provides is teaching and research; anything we might engage in, in the name of service alone, is totally inappropriate. Glenn [Wilson] was clever enough to perceive this, and from his pragmatic, do-it-and-don't-talk-about-it orientation, he still could present this Sunday morning discourse on how this was going to be a wonderful university tool for research.[31]

Wilson's proposal was endorsed; Pickard and team were told to proceed with negotiations with Alston for creating Orange–Chatham. Conant had always been on board with the Orange–Chatham/university partnership. It would provide funding for the Nurse Practitioner Program.

When this all finally came to fruition, Pickard knew that his promise to be in Prospect Hill by spring of 1971 could be met. The university was consumed by the grander scheme for Orange–Chatham, which did include Prospect Hill, and the FNP Program. Quickly, Pickard and McIntyre returned to the drawing board. Margaret Wilkman, who would be in the pilot class, was hired to work with Pickard over the summer to help identify content for the curriculum. Curricular planning could move forward with all seriousness, knowing that, indeed, there would be a program. And student recruitment began in earnest. The funding barrier was checked off the list.

The Capstone

Leadership in the School of Public Health endorsed the nurse practitioner concept. Conant, dean of the School of Nursing, also did—that is why she came to Carolina. That is why she protected the FNP Program. And the dean of medicine was publicly supportive. But as Pickard offered:

> There was no question at that time that Lou Welt was the major power figure within the medical school and anything and everything that you wanted to do within the med school, if Dr. Welt didn't adopt it, you might as well hang it up. [Taylor] was perfectly willing to hear us out when we needed a blessing, but he was not a mover and shaker. Lou Welt was the mover and shaker in the medical school, from my perspective. I don't mean to minimize the importance of having the dean willing to say, "Go for it." But in terms of the converts we really brought along, who were movers and shakers and willing to get things done, Lou was the key.[32]

On many occasions Welt had said that he supported nurse practitioners, primary care in rural areas, etc., but these had been conversational endorsements. He had not made any public pronouncements. Even though he had endorsed the partnership with the Orange–Chatham OEO-funded effort, he had the power to squelch any deal at any time. However, no one expected what happened on the day of the first Kemble lecture.

When Dean Elizabeth Kemble resigned from the School of Nursing, a lectureship fund was established in her honor. She was the founding dean of the School of Nursing and had served as dean for eighteen years. The first Kemble lecture was held in the spring of 1970, in the large auditorium in the new School of Nursing building, Carrington Hall. Several noted with surprise and awe that Welt was participating at this lecture.

Loretta Ford, the originator of the pediatric nurse practitioner initiative from Denver, Colorado, was the featured speaker. Welt participated in the program as well. As Conant described the event:

> I think Loretta Ford's lecture in the spring of '70 was a milestone. Somehow, we persuaded Lou Welt to represent the medical viewpoint. He and Loretta really interacted with each other and had a good time together on the program. There was a good audience, Loretta was convincing to the nurses and [the occasion of the lecture] got issues and possibilities out in the open.... [Welt] kept his word and didn't back out or change his mind. When he said OK to the idea of developing the FNP training program and practice sites, it gave the whole thing life.... Lou Welt is probably one of the unsung heroes.[33]

Booth, in discussion with Pickard, reflected and then asked:

> It might have been one of the first Kemble lectures. I'm not sure what year it was when Loretta Ford came, and Lou Welt gave his endorsing speech. Probably Margaret Dolan might have been involved. I can remember it in the auditorium in the new School of Nursing. Of course, I didn't know Lou Welt had been in on all

these planning meetings. I asked [myself], "Who wrote this speech for him?" Pickard replied, "Who wrote the script? That was his own. I'd forgotten that, because that to me was anticlimactic. But it was a very significant event in terms of a public display of what I perceived to be a battle that had already been won."[34]

The third hurdle had been cleared with aplomb!

MOVING ON

With funding secured and endorsement from the highest levels within the institution, a commitment was made to move forward with a family nurse practitioner program. The hurdles of faculty, funding, and endorsements all came together almost simultaneously in the spring of 1970. The program would start in the fall of 1970. Glenn Pickard, Marie McIntyre, Judy Watkins, Evelyn Aabel, Margaret Wilkman, and others working on the curriculum had to shift into high gear. They had to hustle to develop recruitment plans and admission criteria. And they had about as much time to do all that as it took you to read this chapter!

But there was energy. They had been dreaming and scheming for at least the past five years. As Pickard recalled, "There was just a whole incredible coalescence of events." To him, it was finally clear: "Our [UNC] institutional response was to be the nurse practitioner."[35] And so the Family Nurse Practitioner Program at the University of North Carolina started on September 8, 1970. It was not always easy sailing, but most of the time the movers and shakers felt the wind at their backs.

ADDENDA

Lead Allies toward a New Order of Things

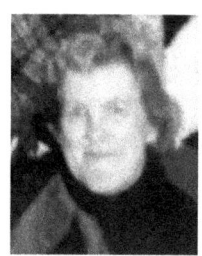

Julia Day Watkins (1928–2012), known as Judy to many, gave steadfast support and leadership to the UNC Family Nurse Practitioner Program from 1970 to 1978. Even before the program began, she supported the idea of a nurse practitioner, working behind the scenes with nurses and physicians from the Schools of Public Health, Nursing, and Medicine. When asked by Margaret Dolan if she should give national voice and support to the nurse practitioner concept, Judy offered wise counsel, encouraging Dolan to do so.

Judy Watkins spent her entire career in public health nursing, and like many public health nurses, she viewed the nurse practitioner role as a natural extension of public health nursing and a way to improve the practice of nursing as well as improve the availability of health care services generally. She saw a different future and headed for it.

When the Nurse Practitioner Program at UNC started in 1970, it needed faculty who were nurses. Judy stepped up. She did any number of endless things to start a new program. Little planning had transpired for the preceptorship period, so Judy took hold and organized content and seminars to be offered during the preceptorship. She also gave structure to site visits that would occur during the preceptorship period. Then she looked ahead and prepared herself to become the director of the program.

First, she went through the program to learn to be a nurse practitioner. As she said, "I'm not going to direct something if I don't fully understand what it is." As director, Judy found herself talking to nurses filled with excitement about the new program and wanting in, and in the next minute talking to some irate physician, or nurse, threatening to do "a, b, or c" to stop this program dead in its tracks. And then in the following

minute she had to deal with young faculty and NPs who wanted everything to move faster than it was and who were not too keen on some of
the political compromises that had to be made to gain legal and professional acceptance of the nurse practitioner.

She managed all the excitement and conflicts as only Judy would—
with grace, aplomb, and a quiet but firm resolve. She stepped up when
few nurses would. She was steadfast in her belief. She was resolute—and
sometimes stubborn (the line between the two can be blurry)—but she
was resolute in defending the Nurse Practitioner Program. She brought a
certain degree of wisdom that the young faculty she worked with lacked.
She was quite tolerant of this new, young breed of faculty in the program;
she was never threatened by them, and gave them their head to try new
things, to branch out. She supported and encouraged this.

Those who worked with Judy have great respect for her as a wise and
resolute woman. She was a woman of gentle spirit, with unshakable
resolve and great courage.

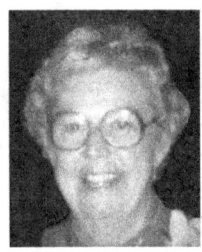

Audrey Joyce Booth (1924–2019). From the dust
bowl of Nebraska, a curly-headed blonde climbed on
a horse twice her height to ride to-and-from a one-
room country schoolhouse, and then ended up as an
associate dean at the University of North Carolina at
Chapel Hill. On her way from that Nebraska farm,
she first went east, stopping at Cleveland, Ohio, to earn one of the early
"direct entry" Master of Science in Nursing degrees. From there, she went
to the far western point of the country, Hawaii (a territory then), with a
stopover in Guam. In 1954, her final cross-country move took Audrey to
a university town near the east coast, Chapel Hill, North Carolina.

This pioneer from Nebraska was a pioneer in many ways. She became
an expert in the care of polio patients during the height of the epidemic

in the '50s, including caring for children in iron lungs. Her expertise took her to Guam and brought her east to UNC. After the polio epidemic, she was the lead nurse in opening the new hemodialysis unit at the VA hospital in Durham, North Carolina, one of the very early dialysis units in the country. Three years later, Audrey joined the North Carolina Regional Medical Program, part of a national health planning effort conceived of as part of President Lyndon B. Johnson's "Great Society" program.

There, Booth served as director of health professions education and held a faculty appointment at the UNC-CH School of Nursing. As described in this book, she was an integral part of the small, select, revolutionary group that commandeered the efforts of many, developing strategies to move the nurse practitioner idea in clinics across the state of North Carolina.

Though highlighting the major steps in Booth's career, that does not, however, represent the essence of Audrey J. Booth as a leader, a role model, and a mentor to many. Her professional life was full of "firsts," and she coached others to become leaders in "first" or innovative efforts as well. In North Carolina alone, likely fifty nurses consider her their mentor—a mentor in the truest sense of that word. Often, she taught by example, the longest-lasting method.

Booth possessed, as well, the courage and ability to lead some of the most contentious and potentially explosive meetings between state leaders in organized nursing and medicine. Those meetings never turned explosive; contentious, yes, but never explosive. Audrey handled strong differences of opinion respectfully and graciously. She was *always* prepared for any meeting, starting a meeting not by asking those present to introduce themselves, but by carefully introducing everyone herself, detailing their background and reason for being present. She thus gave legitimacy and honor to each person present regardless of their position or power. The powerful were not allowed to dominate.

She never misrepresented her position to anyone, be it to friend or foe, and never betrayed an ally, for it is with allies that things get accomplished. Booth was masterful in difficult political situations, a marvel to watch, and giving much to learn if one paid attention.‑

When Audrey Booth retired from her professional career, she did not retire. She always "lived life" fully, not being interested in just passing through. She enjoyed and relished each moment. She took up birding and hooked many of us into her most enjoyable forays into forests, streams, lakes, and wherever else a rare bird made its nest. Her love of nature led her to the Triangle Land Conservancy of North Carolina, where she gave generously of her talents to lead and to raise funds. Audrey was primarily responsible for securing the land that now makes up the 296-acre Johnston Mill Nature Preserve. Its hiking trails are named after birds, and within the preserve a creek branches off, aptly named the "Booth Branch."

From Audrey's eulogy: "Plain and simple: Audrey was an influencer, on a grand scale and with each individual. She was a strong voice for nursing and a strong model for women when women were still fighting for their due recognition and for substantial opportunities to influence policies and to assume leadership roles."[36]

CHAPTER SIX

A New Order Begins: The Pilot Class, Pilot Program, and First NP Clinic

Those who have participated in any new program or pilot class know what it's like—the exciting highs of breaking new ground and the camaraderie that develops among them and their fellow trailblazers. They also recall their fears of joining a new program: "What if this fails? What if I fail?" They remember that some of the details necessary for the new program had not yet been tended to, but at the same time, they look back on how much they learned by helping the new program succeed. And then they value the satisfaction of being a part of its success.

The first class of the Family Nurse Practitioner Program at the University of North Carolina at Chapel Hill was called the "pilot class" as opposed to the "first class." Other programs starting in the early 1970s did the same—often without knowing of each other's naming protocol. It was a face-saving way to address the worrisome question, "What if it fails?" If it failed, they could claim later that it was an experiment. Furthermore, calling it a "pilot" was a way to assuage the faculty who had opposed the nurse practitioner concept, giving them a sense that they might still be able to have some salvaging effect on the next iteration of the program. But most importantly, program proponents had been dreaming of this program for years, yet when it began, they had had little time to plan for it in a way they would have preferred. They knew it would change after the first years' experience and assessment, so they called it a "pilot" to give themselves flexibility to make needed changes and adjustments as they went along and into successive classes. Such latitude was certainly needed given the abridged four to six months of planning time before the program began.

PLANNING ON THE FAST TRACK

On March 11, 1970,[1] Orange–Chatham Comprehensive Health Services, Inc. (OCCHS) incorporated as a joint venture of the University of North Carolina at Chapel Hill Division of Health Affairs and the Orange–Chatham OEO Community Action Agency. OCCHS came into being after the "famous" breakfast meeting in the hospital cafeteria mentioned in the previous chapter, wherein the university agreed to move forward with the joint effort.

The agreed-upon mission of OCCHS was to provide comprehensive health care services and education to all in the community, with emphasis on those who weren't receiving proper health care and who lacked access to services.[2] When fully operational, OCCHS would operate two clinics serving rural Orange and Chatham counties, in Prospect Hill and in Haywood-Moncure, respectively. A third OCCHS clinic would be in Chapel Hill–Carrboro, serving the local population who did not have easy access to primary care from the UNC hospital clinics or the very few private practice physicians in Chapel Hill.

Funding for the new NP clinics through the university–OCCHS partnership, however, although critical, was not the only funding need. Funding for ongoing program support, such as additional faculty, administrative services, and student stipends, were also critical if the program was to continue with a stable source of funding after the pilot class. Dean Conant took it on herself to secure this funding.

Following on the heels of the Physician Assistant (PA) Program at Duke University and the Pediatric Nurse Practitioner Program (PNP) at the University of Colorado, in 1969 the National Center for Health Services Research, within the then Department of Health, Education, and Welfare (DHEW), offered funding for two different types of demonstration projects. One funding stream was for nurse practitioners (which the National Center referred to as PRIMEX programs) and the other was for physician assistants (referred to as MEDEX programs).[3] Conant applied for funding, and the School of Nursing was awarded a PRIMEX grant in 1970—just in time. The UNC School of Nursing was among the first to be awarded a PRIMEX grant, along with Cornell University and the Frontier Nursing Service.[4]

It is important to distinguish between the National Center's grant-funded PRIMEX programs and those family nurse practitioner pro- grams who referred to their educational programs as PRIMEX programs. "PRIMEX" was a term coined by Madeline Leininger, from the University of Washington, to emphasize the expanded role and responsibilities of professional nurses in primary care. The University of Washington thus referred to their family nurse practitioner program as a PRIMEX program.[5] Other programs adopted the titling reference and called their educational programs PRIMEX programs as well.

The University of North Carolina, and others, did not adopt, by intention, the use of the term PRIMEX to describe their educational program. They did not want to engender association with the term "physician extender" or the ongoing debate over the terms "expanded" or "extended" roles. Nor did they want to cause confusion among different types of programs, such as MEDEX, programs to train ex-military corpsmen as physician assistants. UNC decided to simply call their program a "family nurse practitioner" program.

Between 1970 and 1972, the National Center for Health Services Research and Development funded seven PRIMEX projects to prepare and evaluate family nurse practitioners. UNC's program was among the first four programs funded by the National Center's PRIMEX project; three other programs were funded in 1971.[6] Thus, an important and necessary differentiation made here, and throughout the book, occurs between nurse practitioner programs that were funded through the PRIMEX grant program of the National Center for Health Services Research and those family nurse practitioner programs that chose to use the term PRIMEX to refer to their educational programs.[7]

With a funding source to operate a clinic in Prospect Hill, to hire additional faculty, and to secure support for students, planning began in earnest—and a considerable amount of preparation was needed. Specifying admission requirements and student recruitment were paramount. Those would be followed by identifying and organizing the critical elements of the curriculum. All of this had to be accomplished in five months.

It's not that the early NP proponents hadn't thought about these things. They discussed the issues frequently. But their thinking and scheming had been hopes and dreams—until they had funding in hand. Now they had to put their ideas on paper in earnest, outlining a curriculum to guide the first six months of classroom and clinical teaching for the nurse practitioner students.

THE PILOT CLASS

Recruitment

With five months to go, student recruitment was not as difficult as they had presumed, but such a short time in which to accomplish it did cause some anxiety for both program codirectors, Pickard and McIntyre.[8] The first year of the OCCHS–university partnership called for six nurse practitioners for three OCCHS clinics: Prospect Hill, Chapel Hill–Carrboro, and Haywood–Moncure. A seventh nurse practitioner student for the Walstonburg clinic would also join the pilot class as the community of Walstonburg was eager to have a local clinic.

OCCHS provided financial support to students who would eventually work at their clinics; the Health Services Research Center provided support to the student returning to work at Walstonburg. Through the OCCHS–UNC partnership, UNC provided the clinic physician staff and the training program for NPs, and OCCHS provided all the supportive and administrative personnel for the clinics. Initially, because of the very abbreviated recruitment period, all hands were on deck to recruit students because all had a stake in getting the right nurses trained as NPs.

During the Prospect Hill study, interviewers had identified nurses local to Orange County as potential candidates for the pilot program. The local Community Action Program (CAP) offices also queried residents about nurses in the local area, nurses whom residents often consulted when they had health questions. Paul Alston, a Chatham County native and the executive director of the Joint Orange–Chatham Community Action Agency, became the first director of OCCHS. He and his staff were committed to the nurse practitioner model and to making quality health care services available to all. Alston, Pickard, Conant, and Dolan were all on the lookout for potential students. Pickard summarized the recruiting process. "The students had been recruited before August, but not much [before then]. We started in the spring. We'd gotten Betty through the Prospect Hill study.... Sandy Hogan, a black nurse, was recruited from the Carrboro community. June Baise was the Walstonburg nurse recruited by that community."[9]

Hogan, a graduate of Harlem Hospital in New York City, was the only black nurse in the pilot class. She was recruited by Alston, who was committed to finding black nurse practitioner students for the OCCHS clinics. UNC had started to admit black undergraduate nursing students in 1965, so he didn't expect to find many UNC graduates. But he did hope to find a graduate of his university, North Carolina Agricultural and Technical State University (NCA&T), one of the state's historically black universities with a nursing program. He did find a nurse graduate from his university for the second class, and through her he was able to recruit Hogan for the pilot class.

Margaret Dolan influenced two MPH students to join the program, Margaret Wilkman and Ruth Efird. According to Efird, "I was getting my MPH in nursing supervision when Margaret Dolan approached me about applying for [the] new NP Program. I was going to be paid $9,000 to be in the program, and then guaranteed a job in rural health in either Orange or Chatham counties. I was definitely the youngest, as well as a newlywed!"[10] Drs. Arden Miller, Bernard Greenberg, and Earl Seigel, from the School of Public Health's Department of Maternal–Child Health, were supportive of the FNP Program from its inception, so they encouraged Aabel and Collins to enroll in the new program—and several other students after that.

Through various means and connections the initial seven nurses for the pilot FNP class were on board. They didn't have a lot of advance notice, however. Betty Compton had been visited several times during the Prospect Hill Study. She was an ideal candidate for the FNP Program. However, the university people involved in the study didn't want to upset the local community by recruiting her away. Compton described it this way:

> You know Glenn [Pickard], and how he sort of dances around? He doesn't settle down very well. He came in, and I was again feeding the baby or something. They didn't want to ask me pointedly whether I was interested or not, because it might impinge on my plans for going back to the health department to work, and they didn't want to really coerce me in any direction.... [B]y that time, they were talking about the training program, and I thought it was an excellent idea, and I would do all I could do to help. They made about four trips, back and forth.

Finally, Glenn got around to asking me if I would consider being in the class to be trained. They were trying to find out if I was going to stay on the farm, or go back to nursing at the hospital, or to the health department, and I wouldn't commit in any direction. Finally, he said, "We just want to know if you'd like to be in that training program." I said, "You'll have to tell me more about it." When they left, I was elated because I thought it was a super opportunity, and that's what I wanted.

I had a lot of ideas about what we could be doing if we just had the room and the backup to do it. That was maybe August 20, that last visit. The class started on September 8. They needed my credentials quickly, and references and all these things. I know as well as you do, they probably didn't do [much] with them .... They never called, didn't have time. That is how quickly it took place.[11]

Admissions Criteria

Admissions criteria had not been formalized by late spring 1970 when student recruitment needed to begin. However, ongoing discussions about expanding nurses' responsibilities in the continuing care clinic in the hospital as well as in NP-staffed clinics in rural communities provided a general, even if not fully defined, framework for those considering applicants to the new program. The guiding admissions criteria developed for the first pilot class continued to be of use for the next seven to eight years of the program.

Nurses local to the community to be served and known and respected by those communities were of utmost importance in recruiting students during the early years of the program. Program planners did not want NPs coming and going through a revolving door every year or two. In their view, stable nurse practitioner providers were essential for the sustainability of rural clinics. Further, the odds of communities accepting nurse practitioners as their primary care providers would be higher if the NPs were already known to the community.

Another salient criterion for admission was years of clinical nursing experience. Even though nurse practitioners would have formalized relationships and backup support from physicians, many would often be alone in rural clinics. It would not be wise to send novice nurses to isolated rural clinics. Thus, substantial clinical experience also had to be a prerequisite. Initially, program faculty thought public health experience was preferable because public health nurses were accustomed to making independent clinical decisions. However, they later learned that experience in critical/intensive care was also an added benefit—because students from those settings had more knowledge of the pathophysiology of disease and had already learned to function in roles with expanded independent decision-making responsibilities. In the end, both types of clinical backgrounds proved useful.

Another essential criterion was a sponsoring physician, a physician whose practice would provide the student with clinical training during the program's preceptorship phase, and who would be the backup physician for the nurse practitioner after completion of all program requirements. Nurse practitioner advocates had no intention of establishing independent nurse practice sites. They were confident that nurses, with additional training as nurse practitioners, could provide at least 75–80 percent of the primary care needs of communities. But they were just as confident that some situations would require physician consultation, or an in-person physician visit. A backup physician was, therefore, a required component of NP practice. They also knew that such a complementary arrangement would be critical to gaining acceptance of FNPs from the medical community in the state as well.

Program planners felt that nurse practitioners would also alter the practice of physicians, and vice versa. And they felt, too, that the nurse–doctor relationship would change, becoming a collaborative rela-tionship. For the pilot class, the sponsoring-physician criterion was pre-determined as physicians from the university's Community Medicine Division would be working in the OCCHS clinics and would be the sponsoring physicians.

The final criterion for admission was references from known phy-sician and nurse colleagues. Formal written recommendations were required, but they were also followed up by informal conversations and phone calls. In addition, registered nurse licensure in North Carolina was verified. The last step in the admission process was interviews with Pick-ard, McIntyre, Conant, Alston, and other selected university faculty and OCCHS staff.

Specified educational degrees were not a criterion—though this was a hard bone of contention among nursing faculty, both at UNC and across the country. In 1970, however, there was a significant nurse shortage, not because of a decreasing supply, but because of a surge in demand mainly brought about by the new Medicare and Medicaid legislation of the pre-vious decade. Not only was there a shortage of nurses, but those with bac-calaureate degrees were in even shorter supply. Nationally, fully half, 52.4 percent, of all practicing nurses held diplomas in nursing, granted by hos-pital schools of nursing.[12] In North Carolina, the situation was more dire. A 1967 report to the legislature reported in that same year that almost three-quarters, 73 percent, of new North Carolina nurse graduates came from diploma programs. There were only seven baccalaureate programs in the state at the time compared to twenty-six diploma schools.[13, 14] If nurse practitioner programs in the 1970s accepted only nurses with bac-calaureate degrees, rural primary care needs could not be met—especially in North Carolina. Consequently, the nurse supply issue had a significant influence on determining educational criteria for program admission.

Furthermore, most of the physician NP advocates based their

decisions on their experiences with nurses. Just as nurses "know" who the good doctors are, so too do doctors "know" the good nurses. Nurses and doctors who work together clinically get to know each other's skills and strengths, and they respect each other for what each contributes to any situation. The doctors who worked in the continuing care clinic taught nurses from all types of nursing schools expanded skills. They knew that nurses of all types could and did make sound clinical judgments in the community and in patients' homes. They saw no need to make any differentiation for admission to an FNP program based only on educational credentials.

The NP programs in North Carolina were not the only programs that did not require specific educational degrees for program admission. Most of the early NP programs across the country adopted the criteria advocated by the National Center for Health Services Research and Development (NCHSRD, or the National Center) in its PRIMEX Demonstration and Evaluation grant program—which did not specify any required educational background for admission to an FNP program. The National Center's criteria for student admission simply stated that

> The PRIMEX [funded] programs build upon previous academic and professional experience and focus upon the extension of the scope of nurse practice. It is assumed therefore that the trainees (graduate nurses representing all types of education programs) will have competence, in varying degrees, in universally accepted objectives for generalized nursing practice.[15]

However, the debate continued for several years, even though nurse practitioners of different educational backgrounds proved to be successful and competent. This issue continued until most NP programs moved to master's degree programs.

Nonetheless, the admissions criteria initially adopted, commitment to rural practice, plus preferably being from the rural area in which the NP would work, several years of clinical practice, positive references from trusted colleagues, and sponsorship from clinics or physician practices, served as valuable admissions criteria for many years.

Curriculum

Most of the "new" knowledge and skills needed by nurse practitioners was that associated with physician knowledge and skills and/or claimed by physicians as their own. Since there were very few family nurse practitioners, most of the teaching during the early years of the program had to be done by physicians. The physicians who had taught expanded skills to nurses in the continuing care clinic did so informally and one-on-one. The diseases and problems of patients seen in the clinic, and those that needed follow-up at home, defined the content and skills taught. Consequently, a formal curriculum outline was unnecessary in the continuing care clinic. However, with seven new students coming for a five-month combined classroom and clinical training program, a curriculum plan was required.

Pickard said, "We planned the curriculum month by month, week by week."[16] Planning the curriculum and recruiting medical faculty was Pickard's job. During the summer of 1970, Margaret Wilkman shadowed Pickard in the clinic, making notes of all the things they thought needed to be part of the curriculum. Wilkman recalled a small committee meeting, including Evelyn Aabel, Jessie Pergrin, Pickard, and Frank Loda, a pediatrician, to "hash out a curriculum. The medical parts were easy. The nursing part, especially in terms of family dynamics, was agonizing.... There were discussions about reteaching us, as nurses, to do what we ought to do."[17]

Other small groups worked independently to identify what they thought should be in the curriculum. Some of these groups were in the School of Public Health, others in the School of Nursing. Unfortunately, the work of these groups was not a coordinated effort. But, by whatever means, they managed to cross-pollinate their ideas. As Pickard said, "Somehow, we managed to get everything in place along about August 1970."[18] Pickard, always optimistic, was referring not only to the curriculum but also to student recruitment, faculty recruitment, and admissions—the whole program.

Wilkman, alternatively, summarized the curricular work of the summer: "Glenn and I had put together probably enough of a curriculum to cover six weeks, perhaps eight weeks."[19] No matter how much or how little of the curriculum outline was in place, it was enough to start the program. And so, on September 8, 1970, the first nurse practitioner program in North Carolina began.

THE PILOT PROGRAM: OFF AND RUNNING

As noted earlier, there was excitement as well as apprehension among all present on the first day—the seven nurse practitioner students as well as Pickard and Conant. The first day did not follow any curricular plan. Both Conant and Pickard shared their ideas, hopes, and dreams about what nurse practitioners might accomplish. Pickard told them how it all started—how he and his fellow physicians believed nurses could do more than they were currently allowed to do, how NPs would help solve the primary care crisis, and how they hoped to have NP clinics dotted across the state.

Pickard and Conant then talked about how they thought the year would progress. The program was a year-long program, with two phases. The first phase, the on-campus phase, would be in Chapel Hill, consisting of classroom instruction and clinical experiences primarily at North Carolina Memorial Hospital clinics. The second phase, the "preceptorship" phase, would be in the clinics where the future NPs would eventually practice, but they would return to UNC once a month for several days of continued formal instruction.

They also discussed the opposition and downsides of this new endeavor. The students had already experienced resistance to this program from some of their colleagues. But they were unaware of the various medical–legal issues involved, and Pickard told them that the legal parameters of the new role were still unresolved, but this did not deter them. Conant shared her conviction that nurse practitioners would eventually change the practice of nursing—for the better. She knew nurse practitioners would be a game-changer for nursing practice in the future. They all returned the second day, as the pilot group of seven began to coalesce as a group.

The On-Campus Phase

The first weeks of the curriculum focused primarily on physical exams, and gradually moving into physical diagnosis. During this early period, Wilkman recalled:

> We...supported each other in sorting out who we were and what we were; there was a lot of push [effort] within the group,...trying to find security, to come up with a very tight definition of who we were as nurse practitioners.... [In time] there was some sense of who we were and certainly enough sharing of commonality so that we could turn to each other for support, and yet [we had] a very interesting mix of backgrounds.[20]

They also joined forces to help develop the curriculum beyond the first six weeks of planned content. After the first six weeks, the group identified what they needed to learn about common pediatric problems; as overnight assignments, they researched how to diagnose and treat those problems. After discussion, they wrote up what they had learned, and the result of those learning exercises ultimately became pediatric clinical practice guidelines. Wilkman describes what they did:

Each of us would take a disease or two, and we would research the literature, which we would present in class and discuss. Frank [Loda, a pediatric physician] would sort out why things conflicted, where one person would say something, and someone else would disagree. It was tremendous learning.... I see that as one of the best things that happened for the seven of us, and again may have contributed to our becoming very autonomous in the role, because we got to do a lot of ground-level thinking.[21]

No one told the class what to think. They were engaged in active learning. Compton describes this learning/curriculum development process similarly.

We decided somewhere early on in October [1970] that the best way to learn about diseases in pediatrics was to design some sort of a protocol we all would follow. Each of us divvied up the diseases we thought were the most common and that we didn't know how to treat, and then we followed the protocol: the definition, cause, etc. We'd have an assignment on Monday, and when we had pediatrics again on Wednesday, we had to be ready. We really burned a lot of midnight oil.

We did the same thing with symptoms versus disease. We'd take the symptom and do the same thing, asking if you have abdominal pain in a child, what would you be considering? Then Bob [Greenberg, another pediatrician] and Frank Loda would take that and expand on it. That's how pediatrics came about. Then we did some emergency things because we ended up helping with an emergency in pediatrics. We came back and asked, "What should we have done?" I think a lot of the curriculum changed after we opened the clinic when we started to see more patients. It was really shooting from the hip about what should be covered next and to what extent.[22]

Bob (Robert A.) Lawrence came to the School of Medicine in July 1970 and almost immediately found himself in the position of director of professional services for OCCHS. Just as quickly, he jumped into the FNP Program, joining Pickard and Sam Putnam as medical faculty, "teaching sessions for the nurse practitioners who would become my OCCHS colleagues on completion of their training."[23] Lawrence developed a significant portion of the program's adult medicine content, helpful in formalizing the curriculum, particularly for future classes.

The immersion of the pilot class in helping develop curricular content led to their involvement in writing protocols, or patient care guidelines, or standing orders—standards of practice known by various titles. Because the legal standing of NPs was unresolved in 1970, Pickard kept his physician colleagues in the Medical Society and Board of Medicine regularly informed of what they were doing at UNC. No one wanted to raise the suspicion or ire of the professional organization of medicine or the legal body regulating the practice of medicine. Pickard reassured the legal and professional authorities that NP practice was guided by protocols similar to those commonly used in intensive and critical care units (ICUs and CCUs, respectively).

Most ICUs and CCUs opened in the early to mid-sixties in response to increased demand for intensive care and to accommodate new and sophisticated patient monitoring technologies. Physicians were not always available 24/7 in these intensive care units. Therefore, nurses had to be allowed to respond quickly whenever a change in a patient's condition warranted. "Protocols" were established in these ICUs, outlining the circumstances in which nurses could act, often by administering medication according to "standing orders," meaning without a physician's *physician standing orders. Won the precedent for expanded nursing roles*

116   CHAPTER SIX

patient-specific order. Thus, nurses in ICUs were the first to expand their responsibilities. This expansion of function, along with written protocols, had been accepted by practicing physicians and medical–legal authorities. In fact, "physician standing orders" was an accepted practice in medical and surgical units of general hospitals for many years before any expanded nurse role became commonplace.

The use of standing orders in ICUs was not the only stimulus to UNC's development of what it called "patient care protocols." Somewhere in the early curriculum planning phase, a group of interested nursing and medical faculty, including Pickard, visited the Frontier Nursing Service. Most of them knew of the Frontier Nursing Service (FNS) in Kentucky as a horseback-riding midwifery service in Appalachia, started in 1925. But now they also learned that the FNS had expanded its services to include primary care.

horseback riding midwifery

What the North Carolina visitors learned was that the FNS had expanded its services beyond mother and child services, recognizing that more comprehensive services were needed for the entire population in Appalachia. Consequently, the FNS developed "outpost" clinics that were more accessible to those in need—clinics that were like the rural clinics North Carolina was envisioning. The FNS also provided additional informal training to nurses providing comprehensive care services to families in the outpost clinics. Because the nurses would often be alone and far from physicians and other providers, the FNS developed standing orders to guide the nurses in providing care in the outposts.

Pickard looked at the FNS standing orders and took note. This is what we need, he thought, especially for those FNPs who will frequently be on-site alone as the sole provider in many rural clinics. Thus, in the early years it seemed reasonable to use an approach similar to that used in ICUs and at the Frontier Nursing Service to guide and authorize the practice of nurse practitioners. As it turned out, this adaptive approach was frequently an important factor in easing the concerns of practicing physicians who were concerned about quality of care and legal authorization of FNP practice.

The pilot class was instrumental in formalizing what became known as "patient care guidelines." Ruth Efird recalls that "the first patient care protocols [were] written with the first chapter done by the seven of us in my dining room in Married Student Housing."[24] The first chapter of *Patient Care Guidelines for Nurse Practitioners* was titled "Health Maintenance"—the bread and butter of public health nurses. This chapter outlined health maintenance assessments appropriate for different age groups from two weeks to seventeen years. Subsequent chapters identified the majority of health problems encountered in a primary care setting, presenting commonly accepted criteria for diagnosing and managing those common health problems. In the acknowledgments section of the first edition, the authors recognize

> the first class of family nurse practitioners of the University of North Carolina at Chapel Hill: Evelyn Aabel, June Baise, Betty Compton, Ruth Efird, Sandra Hogan, Phoebe Hood, and Margaret Wilkman. As part of their course, they developed a set of pediatric patient care guidelines that served as a foundation for part of this book.[25]

The guidelines were used not only as protocols for clinical practice but also as a curricular structure for subsequent classes of the FNP Program. Many NP practice sites across the state adopted the guidelines, revised them as needed to reflect current practice standards, and adapted them to the unique needs of different practice sites and locations. The guidelines served as a broad set of criteria by which to assess the quality and effectiveness of any NP practice.

The End of the Doctor–Nurse Game

An early lesson beyond learning new physical exam and diagnostic skills was changing how they as nurses related to physicians. The physicians involved in the development of this new role were determined to end the convention of nurses calling their physician colleagues "Dr. so-and-so." To those physicians, such a convention only served to confirm hierarchical differences between doctors and nurses; it did not encourage a collaborative relationship. They told the nurses they would call them "Betty," "Margaret," "Phoebe," etc., not Mrs. Compton or Ms. Betty. And they expected that the nurses would call them Glenn, Frank, Bob, Harvey, Zel, etc. Pickard would say, "No more me Tarzan, you Jane."

This was not always easy for the pilot seven. They would forget, or fall into old habits, or just couldn't find their comfort level with a new manner of addressing physicians. The physicians were persistent, though. They decided that whenever they were addressed as Dr. so-and-so, they would simply ignore the comment or question, as if they hadn't heard it. Finally, everyone caught on—first-name basis only.

The issue of salutation may appear superficial today. But it was far from that in 1970. The tradition of more formal salutations was emblematic of the status and power differentials between nurses and physicians. It also mirrored the issues raised by the women's movement of the time, especially since most nurses were female and most physicians were male. The physicians were most adamant about how nurses and doctors were going to address each other—because how they addressed each other would reflect and emphasize how they saw each other. In some situations, nurses knew more about patient care than physicians; in other situations, physicians knew more about patient care. It was a matter of respect for each other's knowledge that would benefit a patient, and never one type of practitioner being better than the other. In 1970, it was a huge step forward in changing how nurses and physicians saw each other and related to each other, and above all, prioritized patient benefit.

The Preceptorship Phase

No predetermined end date had been set for the on-campus portion of the program for the pilot class. When the faculty thought they were ready, they said: let's move into the preceptorship phase. The NP students received their certificates of program completion in December 1970, but still had to finish the preceptorship. Ideally, or at least according to the plan, NP students would return to their "sponsoring" clinic for their preceptorship. The purpose of the preceptorship was to give students additional, more intensive hands-on clinical experience in their new role and also to give them and their backup physicians time to establish a new and different type of working relationship.

For June Baise, the path was quite clear. She would return home to finish her preceptorship with a physician in private practice in Wilson, North Carolina—in preparation for the new clinic in Walstonburg. Baise did finish the preceptorship. However, she never went to work at the Walstonburg clinic as her husband's job required a transfer, so they both moved from eastern North Carolina to another part of the state. As it turned out, the Walstonburg clinic would not be ready for another two years—giving the community time to recruit another NP for the clinic.

For the other six students, the plan for the next six months was a little murky. They knew they were committed to OCCHS. But OCCHS had a short start-up period, just as the FNP Program had. Incorporated in March 1970, OCCHS had little time to get three clinics up and functional within a year. Then, too, they didn't receive their first start-up grant from the Office of Economic Opportunity until July 1970. Although they hoped to open in less than a year, the likelihood of such lessened

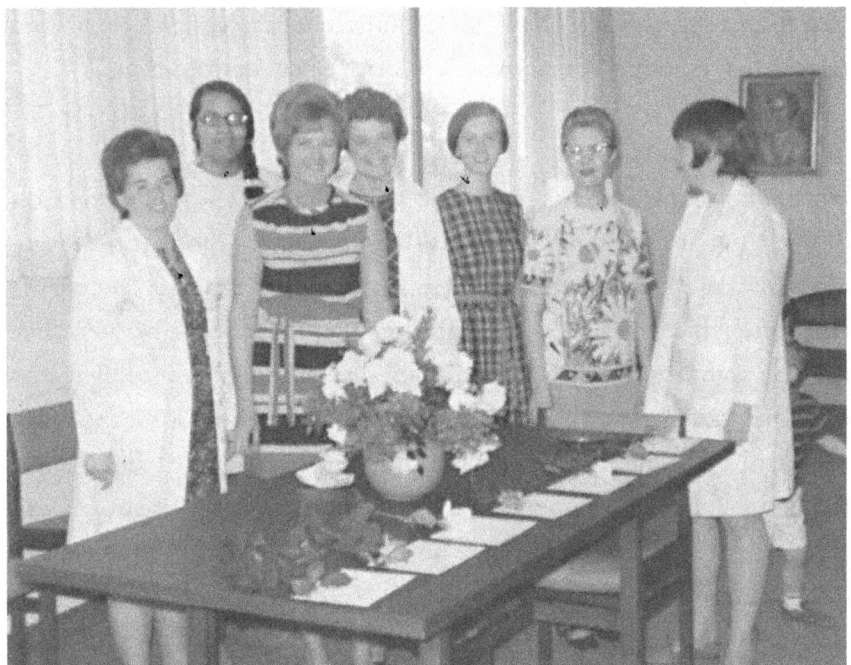

FNP pilot class graduates after receiving certificates. From left to right: Betty Compton, Sandra Hogan, Phoebe (Hood) Collins, Evelyn Aabel, Ruth Efird, June Baise, and Margaret Wilkman. (Hiding behind Wilkman is Efird's toddler.)

daily. A clinic building was ready for occupancy in Prospect Hill, but there were no buildings in Carrboro or Moncure—the planned locations of the other two clinics. Having three clinics spanning the Chatham and Orange County service areas was the grand plan. As it turned out, however, the Prospect Hill clinic opened in July 1971; the Carrboro clinic followed later in 1971, but services were offered in rental space in Chapel Hill until a new building was completed; and the Moncure clinic did not begin seeing patients until April 15, 1972.

In addition to a building, the physical structure to house a clinic, trained staff were also required. Office staff, including medical records staff, were needed, as were clinic assistants, lab technicians, and community health workers. Recruitment and training of personnel were of the highest priority, and equipping clinics was the next big step—no small order. No wonder clinic openings were delayed. Once again, the program faculty and coordinators had to be quick to arrange alternate preceptorship experiences for the six OCCHS students until their designated clinics could open.

The OCCHS/UNC partnership agreement called for two to three UNC physicians to provide medical backup support at each of the OCCHS clinics. The program faculty wanted to pair each NP student with the physicians they would ultimately work with at the OCCHS clinics. The initial OCCHS internists were Glenn Pickard, Zel (Axalla) Hoole, Edward Wagner, and Sam Putnam. They were willing to serve as preceptors for the FNP students, but how would they fit the students into the already oversubscribed clinics at the hospital? As it was, medical students, interns, and residents were falling over each other as they all tried to learn by seeing patients in the clinics.

With the start of the FNP Program and the anticipation of local OCCHS clinics, the continuing care clinic phased out to incorporate the FNP students' preceptorship experiences. Students alternated rotations in the revamped continuing care clinic, now the general medicine clinic. Pediatric experiences were provided in the pediatric clinics with Sid Chapman, Harvey Hamrick, Frank Loda, and Fred Summers.

In some ways, none of the six FNPs had what might be called an "ideal" preceptorship. It was more of a patchwork preceptorship, crafting together a variety of necessary and fascinating experiences. At the same time, their unusual preceptorships gave them clinical experiences they might not have had in a new primary care setting. By the end of April, they were ready to leave the guiding arm of the program to begin working as family nurse practitioners. Those FNPs assigned to the Prospect Hill clinic went to that newly opened clinic. Since the other two OCCHS clinics were either operating at reduced capacity in rental space or the clinic buildings were not yet built, the four other OCCHS FNPs rotated between the temporary Chapel Hill clinic and the Prospect Hill clinic.

The Insurance Issue

Once the preceptorship period was underway, Pickard and other doctors knew they had to sort out the liability issue. Glenn Wilson knew this was critical, based on his experience starting other clinics. However, none of them knew whether the liability insurance available to nurses would cover them in their new expanded role. Nor did they know if, as nurse practitioners working with a specific physician, the physician's liability insurance would cover a nurse practitioner's liability. But they had a sense that most physicians would not want to incorporate another provider under their own liability insurance. They had to find an insurer for these new nurse practitioner health providers.

Pickard, Booth, Wilson, and others had attended a national conference in 1969 sponsored by Duke University on the legal status of the physician assistant (PA). Clark Havinghurst and David Warren, two notable health law attorneys, spoke. Although the discussion focused on PAs, it was relevant to similar issues NPs faced. As Pickard noted, " [We] came out of the [conference] with the resolve that if this was going to fly very far, it had to be legitimized. One of the key things in terms of legitimization was Wilson's belief that he didn't care whether it was legal; it had to be insurable."[26]

Glenn Wilson knew the insurance industry and its leaders well from his past experiences. He got the attention of the St. Paul Companies, Inc., hereafter referred to as St. Paul's. It was the largest underwriter of medical malpractice insurance in the country at the time. He arranged to have the top leadership of St. Paul's and their underwriters and actuarial professionals visit Chapel Hill. Before they visited, Wilson, Pickard, (David) Warren,[27] and others prepped. As Pickard described their discussions:

It was first insurable, and then it had to be legal. I remember Glenn [Wilson] beat on Dave Warren and the phrase that Dave came up with was he would tell the St. Paul's people it was not illegal. He kept saying, "Glenn, I can't tell them it's legal." [Wilson] said, "Well, I don't give a damn if you tell them it's legal. Tell them it's not illegal." That was the phrase that we used in many forums. They'd say, "Is this legal?" and we'd say, "The question of legality has not been totally resolved, but we have it from our legal counsel that it's not illegal."[28]

Visionaries- revolutionaries

St. Paul's leadership came. Convinced of the soundness of the nurse now practitioner model, they agreed to provide insurance. The original premium, in 1970, for nurse practitioner liability insurance was eleven dollars a year.

Informing the Medical Society, Nursing Associations, and Professional Boards

As Pickard noted, "[T]hey had the belief that this [nurse practitioner practice] had to get into the mainstream, that it was not something you wanted to hide under the table."[29] They kept all the leaders of the North Carolina Medical Society and North Carolina Nurses Association informed, and, as importantly, the licensing boards for both medicine and nursing. Pickard knew Bryant Galusha and David Citron, members of the Board of Medical Examiners. According to Pickard,

Bryant was the contact person. We went to him in private and said, "Look, this is what we want to do. We really know these people, [they're] going to be practicing medicine, they're going to be making medical diagnoses, and we're not asking you to approve it. We're not officially asking you for any opinion. We just want to tell you we're doing it, and if anybody comes to the Board of Medical Examiners and says, these nurses are practicing medicine, you can say what you wish. We would hope you might say, 'Yes, I know about it. The board has been informed and we're keeping an eye on it, we're following it along,' some such rubric. We know we can't ask you to approve it, and we don't want you to approve it. We don't even want you to officially consider it. Just be knowledgeable and run interference for us."[30]

Ed Beddingfield was aware of the nurse practitioner concept developing at UNC because of his contact with Cecil Sheps, who had talked to him and others in the group practice in Wilson. None of the other physicians in the Wilson clinic had any interest in NPs—except for Beddingfield. He knew full well that many of his fellow North Carolinians were without adequate health care, and he believed nurse practitioners could help alleviate their problems. Being new to the group practice, Beddingfield did not wield much influence with his physician colleagues. But he was an up-and-coming leader in the North Carolina Medical Society and would eventually become its president. Pickard, Sheps, Booth, and others made sure that crucial leaders like him were informed about the experiment taking place at UNC.

On the nursing side, Lucy Conant and Audrey Booth reached out to the Board of Nursing. The nursing board did not have jurisdiction over continuing education programs offered by schools of nursing, and consequently the nurse practitioner role was not, at that time, a legal concern of the Board of Nursing. However, all those involved in starting the Nurse Practitioner Program knew they needed to be on prevention alert. They wanted to establish trusting relationships with nursing's professional and legal organizations. They set out to inform the leaders of these organizations about what they were doing. If any questions arose among their constituency, they wanted those leaders to come directly to them with their issues.

Margaret Dolan of the School of Public Health ensured that the leadership of the North Carolina Nurses Association was up to date. She had served as its president and was highly respected. Her commitment to the nurse practitioner movement and her influence in the nursing association was unquestionably helpful in allaying the opposition of many in nursing.

Audrey Booth was positioned strategically at the North Carolina Regional Medical Program, as director of health professions education. In her role, she frequently interacted with nurse and physician leaders in the state. She was a boundary spanner among many groups and was in a unique position to advocate or clarify whenever necessary, providing an informative report about the developing program at UNC. As importantly, she could strategically make others aware of nurse practitioners and their positive impact on services in North Carolina. Booth was well situated; she could learn about any potential or developing pockets of resistance so that key members of the planning group could mitigate problems that might arise—before they became major issues. She was actively involved with the North Carolina Nurses Association, and would soon be appointed to serve on the North Carolina Board of Nursing and eventually become its chair.

Pickard, Conant, Dolan, and Booth were not only staunch advocates of the nurse practitioner; they were also astute politicians. Their careful watch over the concerns of the professional bodies was critical during the early phases of the nurse practitioner movement. The relationships they developed during the first years proved to be monumentally crucial during the three to five years following the pilot program.

THE FIRST NP CLINIC

While Wilkman and Compton were finishing their preceptorships, Alston and his staff recruited clinic staff, focusing on the Prospect Hill clinic as they knew this would be the first clinic to open. The first NP clinic opened in July 1971 in Prospect Hill. As Wilkman recalls,

We expected when we opened the clinic that we would probably sit on our hands for months, and we expected that people would come in and kind of test the water and see what-was-what. For a month, I think less than two weeks.... And they flocked in. We opened in July with no equipment and untrained people as support. Betty and I, with Martha Garst [of OCCHS], began to develop a curriculum for training community health workers and nursing assistants and clinic assistants, this kind of stuff. This finally came to fruition in September or October, but meanwhile Betty and I, off the top of our heads, [were] doing all of the basic training to get the thing up and going in Prospect Hill.[31]

Geneva Warren was also worried about how the community would accept the clinic. She worried about how people "used to being doctored to by a man" would respond to female nurse practitioners. Geneva (Warren) and Glenn (Pickard), watching from Geneva's house across the road, were keyed up when the clinic opened. Geneva tells the story:

In the first place, I hate to admit this, but today it's nice, and it's fun, and it's great when the two races come together, and it's nothing. But Glenn and I were quaking in our boots and opened a bottle of Champagne here in this room when all the people who were involved in the clinic [gathered] over there, and there's about a 50–50 sort of thing, you know. And we didn't know how that was going to hit as far as the community was concerned.... But just as all of us have thankfully and in our own innards known, it was the right thing; it came along very well. But the citizenry of the whole community is quite proud.

After all, when you realize that the clinic was built with two

separate waiting rooms, one for the black and one for the white—
or certain of the community would not support it. That was a stipulation of some of the people who felt so strongly that way. Well, we
still didn't know how that was going to come along, and then, too,
how they were going to feel about [being seen by] women initially.

But I knew we had it made when Mr. Hub Long down here at
the store said, "Well, I went out there. I didn't know how it was
going to be." And he said, "The woman told me to undress," and
he said, "I didn't know about that, but before we got through, I
felt like I was examined from the bottom of my feet to the top
of my head. She took plenty of time with me. I liked the way she
talked, and it wasn't bad. I just believe it's going to be all right." He
was a fairly elderly man, and it usually takes somebody younger to
adjust; I felt like we were well on the way.[32]

The issue of race and separatism, in health care, was quietly resolved
by assimilation in this rural community. When the clinic building was
planned in the fifties, there were to be two waiting rooms, one for white
people and one for black people. That was the stipulation of many white
people who donated money for the clinic; that was the way it was in the
fifties in the South. But racial segregation, by signage and physical design,
was slowly dissipating.

For sure, the university and OCCHS, an OEO outgrowth, would
have it no other way. Segregated waiting rooms would be a thing of the
past; there would be only one waiting room. Indeed, the Prospect Hill
clinic was on its way. They got so busy seeing patients and training staff
that Ruth Efird and Phoebe Collins were often sent to Prospect Hill to
help out while they waited for their clinic in Moncure to open. The Prospect Hill community welcomed nurse practitioners.

The Board of Medicine Visits

Once the clinic opened officially, Pickard told Bryant Galusha, chair of the Board of Medical Examiners, that he should come to see the clinic for himself. Pickard anticipated that Galusha might pay a visit once the clinic opened. Galusha wanted to support the clinic and NPs and thought he should have some firsthand knowledge. Galusha did make that visit, which is best described in the words of both Pickard and Compton. From Pickard:

> So, [Galusha] decided he'd come pay a visit. He came trundling up to the clinic, and I went to the front door to greet him. About that time, an ambulance pulled into the side parking lot, and I was standing there thinking, "Oh, God, what in the hell is this? He's going to yank my chain now." And yet, just with complete aplomb, I introduced him to all the people and started through the clinic, showing him the waiting room and the record room and—. Yes, just thinking, "Oh, God. What are they doing?"
>
> I opened the door, and there was Betty [and Margaret], and this black man—what in the devil? [Name redacted], I guess, was his name. Anyhow, he was an older black man who had gotten up from the table that morning and fallen over, allegedly had a seizure. The family called the rescue squad, and they hustled him into the clinic. Betty got him up on the table, and he looked cold and clammy, a little bit green around the gills, but there was no clue as to what had gone wrong. She took his blood pressure, and it was just barely palpable. She'd gotten an IV started when he proceeded to wolf up a liter of blood. He'd had an occult GI bleed from an ulcer and bled into his stomach; that's what had caused the seizure.
>
> She had all this sorted out and well managed when he [Galusha] opens the door and says, "Well, what's going on here?" Ms.

Compton said, "Well, this man," thus and so. "We have an IV running," and here's the rescue squad. You couldn't have staged it better in a million zillion years. He still remembers that to this day, as do I and everybody else, and he still thinks we staged it.[33]

From Compton:

What he [Pickard] did was he got to Bryant Galusha and convinced him that he needed to see what it was like, if he really wanted to find out if we were what he said, and so forth. A very unannounced, unplanned drop-in visit—he actually flew in here from Charlotte and was put in a car and brought to Prospect Hill, totally unannounced to Margaret and me. We had this dramatic emergency that couldn't have been better timed, that took place in the back, in the trailers, in the first room on the left. It was a patient of Glenn's who was asthmatic, dependent on prednisone, who had collapsed on the floor unconscious.

What was happening with our door closed—they were standing outside—you know how you can hear through the walls. Glenn and Bryant [Galusha] were standing there. We were talking. They were about to knock on the door and introduce him, and we were talking about his GI bleed from prednisone, and let's start an IV, and what would you start—it was like this terribly intellectual, smart-sounding conversation. Glenn said he was sitting out there just a' bursting: listen to those two in there just going to town, demonstrating the best. His very key point is that the emergency that happened can be monitored. What was really happening is that one of us had the chart and the other one was busy. Thinking with both heads. We had already called in the rescue squad, so behind him comes the rescue squad, stretcher, and they go in.

We were telling the rescue squad what had happened and that we would contact Dr. Pickard, but that in the meantime, we had an IV going, and we'd ride with them. He was not in shock now, but he had been. We thought it was a GI bleed, etc. Glenn was about to die to get the chart in his hand; he said he couldn't stand not having the chart. But it couldn't have been timed better. It ended up with exactly that being the problem, and that couldn't have happened better. He [Galusha] actually called here to find out what was wrong with the gentleman and how he did and so forth and so on. Bryant didn't stay and talk with us five minutes; he didn't have a tour; he just spent a few minutes and left. We couldn't have done it better. If we didn't handle any more GI bleeds right, that was the one to do. That's how he really became one of our strong supporters in medicine. He's the one who invited us to the medical society meeting and asked me to come down to talk to the group and be on panels; he became a real supportive person.[34]

Betty later, wanting to correct the record, added, "Margaret Wilkman was just as central to that event as I was, because she was the primary in that incident as far as I am concerned."[35]

The Medical Board was now fully informed and supportive. Nurse practitioners would need full legitimization at some point, and that would come in the future. The Prospect Hill clinic was a fully functioning rural community clinic. The Chapel Hill–Carrboro clinic opened with OCCHS renting space in the outpatient department of the UNC hospital. Efird and Collins continued to work in both the Chapel Hill–Carrboro and Prospect Hill clinics until their clinic opened in the spring of 1972. The demonstration (i.e., the pilot program) was considered a success, and plans to continue more NP classes and clinics moved ahead.

CHAPTER SEVEN

The Next Few Years: Beyond the Pilot Class

As the pilot class progressed through the on-campus portion of the program and into the preceptorship, faculty knew the "pilot" program was a success. The nurses in the pilot class came with the expected background and knowledge, and they had mastered their new learnings. Others were already inquiring about admission to the program the next time it was offered. From this point forward, the program would be ongoing. It was time for the program directors to turn their attention to the next class, especially to expanding enrollment.

THE FIRST AND SECOND CLASSES

Though the pilot class of 1970 prepared just six nurse practitioners for OCCHS clinics and a single nurse practitioner for the Walstonburg clinic, the following year's class—the first official class—enrolled twelve students. Five additional nurses for OCCHS clinics entered the 1971–72 class,[1] and three students would go to Wake Memorial Hospital in nearby Raleigh.[2] During the mid-sixties, the School of Medicine had established working relationships with several nearby hospitals to expand student clinical experiences and ease referral pathways to and from UNC. Because of these connections, Wake Memorial Hospital asked for three student placements in the 1971–72 class.

But interestingly, word of the new Nurse Practitioner Program spread even farther in North Carolina. One student came from a private practice in Mt. Airy, North Carolina—a small rural community north of Winston-Salem near the Virginia border and close to the Appalachian Mountain range, a town best known as the birthplace of Andy Griffith. Two other students represented a private group practice in Pinehurst, North Carolina. The twelfth student was sponsored by the Western Carolina Developmental Center, a state-operated center for developmentally challenged children and adults in western North Carolina.[3]

The first FNP class was more diverse than the first pilot class in terms of the types of practice settings to which the nurse practitioners would eventually return. However, they all met the admission criteria established early on. Students were registered nurses in North Carolina, indigenous to their local areas, with sponsoring physicians who would provide six-month clinical preceptorships and employment after program completion. Although some of these nurses were not explicitly going to sites in rural areas, they nonetheless would be serving in primary care shortage areas. But, more importantly, nurses coming to the FNP Program during the early '70s were all risk takers. They wanted to expand their clinical practice responsibilities and join an exciting new movement; in that, they were very similar to those in the pilot class.

Marjorie Land reflected on her decision to become a nurse practitioner:

> I could not have fantasized a more perfect career ladder for this thirty-something-year-old wife, mother, and nurse who started too poor to even dream of advanced schooling. Mr. Alston wanted nurses from his alma mater, North Carolina A&T State University, and from his community to be in classes from the beginning. I wanted the same. I asked him to include me when he got his program together, and he did.[4]

Glenda Oldham Hargraves described a similar experience:

My journey began at Orange–Chatham Comprehensive Health Service as an excited nurse of fifteen years, embarking upon a new concept: nurse practitioner. This was truly an intoxicating idea. Blazing new trails has always been a part of my "being." There were challenges, but the ones foremost in my mind were the patients' perceptions of and their acceptance of this new concept, and of me.[5]

On occasions, Hargraves sensed that some preferred not to be seen by her because she was a person of color. On one such occasion after a visit, she overheard the patient stop a physician to ask if this, her prescription, was the appropriate treatment. The physician, unaware of Hargraves's presence, said, "If she examined you and wrote you a prescription for treatment, then it's appropriate." Hargraves noted, "With a smile, I retreated to my office."[6]

During the early years of the program, admissions were carefully screened and limited to those judged to have the greatest likelihood of success in the nurse practitioner role. High visibility rendered them eminently vulnerable to scrutiny and challenges. Thus, continued, and future, acceptance of nurse practitioners, by other health care providers and patients, depended on the momentum and recognition generated by the early demonstrations and practice sites, and nurse practitioners. At the same time, nurse practitioners had to deal with issues of color and segregation in North Carolina during the '70s, but they did not retreat from these issues for the sake of acceptance of the role of NPs. White NPs took care of patients of color and NPs of color took care of white patients. None of the new clinics had separate black and white waiting rooms, a departure from the usual practice only a few years ago. And there were no distinctions made between the haves and have-nots. The

OCCHS clinics honored their mission to provide comprehensive care to all people, including the needy and disenfranchised.

The pilot class had admitted seven students; the first class admitted twelve students. In 1972, twenty students comprised the second class. Although increasing class size from seven to twelve and then to twenty may appear small, the increase was significant for a program that many opposed, and some even questioned its viability. In 1972, OCCHS sponsored only three students, and one of those was Judy Watkins—a nursing faculty member who coordinated the program's preceptorship. At this time, it was clear that Marie McIntyre would serve only one more year as program codirector, and Watkins would step into her position when she completed the training program.

Students in the third class came from the eastern and western parts of the state, as well as from the central Piedmont. And they came from private medical practices, hospital-affiliated clinics wanting to expand their service areas to underserved patients, community centers, child development centers, and other practice sites. One student in the third class came from an urban area, Charlotte, the largest city in the state. The admissions committee was hesitant about this application because it challenged the program's commitment to underserved rural areas. Furthermore, the grants obtained by the program to provide stipends to students were based on the "from rural area, return to rural area" principle adopted to benefit the rural underserved.

Agnes Binder (Weisiger) applied from a private internist's practice in Charlotte. She applied to the program but heard nothing in response. She finally called the program office and inquired about the status of her application. She and her physician backup were able to convince the admissions committee that there were underserved areas in Charlotte, even though it was an urban area. The admissions committee did not have any problem with her credentials and the practice setting; the issue was that they were unable to provide her with a stipend while she attended the program. When the practice told the program that Binder did not need a stipend, she was fully admitted.[7]

After Binder's admission, more nurses from private practices were admitted as were those from the state's larger cities, such as Raleigh, the state's second largest city. Practice settings utilizing nurse practitioners became more diverse, but during the first seven to eight years of the program, most nurse practitioners did return to underserved rural clinics and doctor's offices. Over these years, the original three prototype communities expanded their service areas significantly.

A Side Trip

Note to Reader: In this short section, as the primary informant, I move to first-person narrative.

Coincidental with the admission review for the first class, a UNC graduate student working with Glenn Pickard in the continuing care clinic wanted to enter the FNP Program, incorporating the NP classes and clinical experiences into her graduate studies. Glenn Pickard knew firsthand the energy and advocacy this student would bring to the NP movement, and he wholeheartedly endorsed this idea. Faye Pickard, the student's faculty advisor, also supported this notion. Both Pickards, and Conant, had envisioned that the NP Program would ultimately be a graduate-level offering. I was that student.

The first hurdle was gaining approval for the NP classes and preceptorship as alternative experiences for the required graduate clinical courses. If approved, graduate course credit could be awarded for the twelve months of study in the NP Program. The second hurdle was getting approval from Paul Alston and the staff of OCCHS—as one of the OCCHS clinics would provide the sponsoring physician, namely Pickard, and the practice site.

Neither hurdle was an easy jump. Earning graduate course credit for the NP classes and clinical experiences required the School of Nursing graduate faculty's approval. As described earlier, most faculty were opposed to the NP Program. They suspected that resources intended for the school's undergraduate and graduate programs were being diverted to the NP Program. Further, they held the opinion that the entire notion of the nurse practitioner was not good for nursing.

Betty Sue Johnson was a vocal opponent of the NP concept—and as director of the graduate program in the School of Nursing, she wielded considerable influence. Despite Faye Pickard's advocacy for the proposal to grant graduate course credit, the graduate faculty did not support the plan. Besides, Paul Alston and other OCCHS staff were not in favor of the proposal either. They feared that a graduate student from the North like me would not honor a one-year commitment to practice in North Carolina. For these reasons, it was not until 1978 that a pathway for nurse practitioner training at the graduate level was offered.

I was disappointed, but my interest in the NP Program and movement persisted. I continued to work with Glenn Pickard in the UNC clinics, gaining as much informal NP training as possible. "No-show" appointments provided time for Pickard and me to discuss many of the issues surrounding the NP movement in North Carolina, particularly the professional, university, and community political conflicts. In these conversations, Pickard and I talked about how I could fulfill my graduate thesis requirement by studying the new nurse practitioners. I reviewed previous studies to date; most were descriptions of various demonstration projects across the country. I also talked to the nurses and physicians involved in the NP Program at UNC.

Two questions seemed important during the first two years of the program. One was to determine what proportion of a nurse practitioner's practice involved more customary medical activities versus long-established nursing activities. Such information would address whether nurse practitioners were more like mini-doctors or whether their role was a blend of nursing and medicine, reflecting the changing boundaries of nursing and medical practice.

The second study goal was to assess how often nurse practitioners consulted with their backup physician, and in turn, how often the backup physician consultations resulted in a referral to a specialist. These latter measures would provide validation of the assumption that nurse practitioners can provide primary care services to most patients seeking such care, and that nurse practitioners can do so with an appropriate level of physician consultation. The study site was one of the first NP clinics in North Carolina.

I solicited the help of another graduate student (Patricia Merwin) to collaborate on the proposed study. With two investigators collecting data, the study population would be more extensive, and the results more robust.[8,9] The purpose here is not to report on the study findings—other than to say that the assumptions about nurse practitioner practice were confirmed. NPs could manage the vast majority (around 75–80 percent) of primary care patients without physician consultation, and NPs were not functioning as mini-doctors. Their merger of "care and cure" functions were virtually seamless. In their mind and actions, they were both nurses and nurse practitioners, nothing else. Ten years later, Michael Yedidia, in his study of the work of nurse practitioners, also concluded that nurse practitioners do unite cure and care functions within their practice.[10] The study by the two graduate students, Merwin and me, was the first formalized study of nurse practitioners in North Carolina.

REVISITING THE THREE COMMUNITY PROTOTYPES

Prospect Hill, Carrboro, and Moncure: OCCHS Clinics

In the first three years of the program, fourteen nurse practitioners were sponsored by the OCCHS clinics—providing approximately five nurse practitioners for each of the three OCCHS clinics. Almost ten years before the first class of FNP students was admitted, the citizens of Prospect Hill began their search for a physician to replace their beloved family doctor. With a clinic building already in place in Prospect Hill, it was the first of the three OCCHS clinics to open. Prospect Hill welcomed, finally, in the spring of 1971, nurse practitioners and physicians to provide services in the new clinic where many of the pilot and first classes of students worked at some point.

While the second class was in the on-campus phase for classroom and supervised clinical instruction, the Carrboro OCCHS clinic moved from space rented at UNC Hospital to a downtown office building to wait for a new building in Carrboro. With an increasing patient census, more space was necessary, but the Carrboro clinic also needed more visibility and presence in the community it was serving, and the move out of UNC Hospital facilitated that. The same year, the Moncure clinic in Chatham County was also being constructed, opening April 15, 1972—around the midpoint of the preceptorship. That year, 1972, the five students slated for OCCHS had up-and-running clinics to go to, although they did rotate among all three clinics—Prospect Hill, Carrboro, and Moncure—which they felt was an enriching experience as each clinic was unique in many ways. OCCHS was a quickly expanding enterprise, and every year after that the health system sponsored several NP students.

Walstonburg Community Health Center

Cecil Sheps had learned from community leaders in Greene County of their need for health services and their interest in finding a physician. Sheps introduced them to the concept of nurse practitioners, and they sponsored a nurse from the area to enroll in the first pilot class of nurse practitioners. Both Sheps and the Greene County community leaders were eager to get started. The Walstonburg nurse did complete the NP Program, but unfortunately, she moved right after that with her husband as he transferred to another part of the state.

At the same time, despite this loss, something bigger developed in Walstonburg. James (Jim) Bernstein came to Chapel Hill in the fall of 1970 as a Global Health Fellow and began working with Cecil Sheps in the Center for Health Services Research. Walstonburg was a perfect match, an ideal case study for Bernstein because his goal was to provide technical assistance to help communities organize and operate their local health care services, and he did just that in Walstonburg. He helped form a community board, and they, in turn, raised money to build a clinic. But they couldn't find a local nurse to send to the Nurse Practitioner Program. They had to find someone from outside the local area.

Serendipitously, Loretta Ford, founder of the Pediatric Nurse Practitioner Program in Denver, Colorado, was a featured speaker at a UNC School of Nursing conference. Ford met Jessie Pergrin, a School of Public Health student working with Bernstein in Walstonburg. Pergrin told her about her work in Walstonburg, and their need for a nurse practitioner in the Walstonburg community. Ford had a person in mind for the job. As Donna Schafer recalls:

> You know how I heard about Walstonburg? I was still in Colorado in graduate school, kind of getting restless and looking for something new and exciting to do. Lee [Loretta] Ford came to Chapel Hill for a research conference.... Lee came back; she had met Jessie Pergrin. She probably knew of her before, but it was the first time she had ever met Jessie. Jessie told Lee about this community she was working with in the eastern part of the state that was looking for a nurse practitioner. Lee and Jessie thought maybe I would fit what they wanted, so Lee came back and told me about

it. Jessie called me shortly after. And then I went to North Caro-
lina at Christmas time while I was on a break in graduate school.
I remember Jessie meeting me at the airport, and I also remember
Jim and Sue Bernstein meeting me at the airport.[11]

Schafer met with the NPs at Prospect Hill—Compton and Wilkman.
She also met with Pickard, Conant, and Sheps, and then Bernstein took
her to Walstonburg to meet with Beddingfield, who would be the backup
physician for the clinic, and with the executive committee of the Walstonburg Community Board. Schafer describes this meeting.

Yes, with the executive committee. Allen Edwards was the chairman at that time. We were at his house, and four people—he and
the vice chairman, secretary, and treasurer—I think about four
people and their families. We just sat and chatted. I remember
Early Lang, who was the treasurer, telling me that the main things
that they grew in North Carolina were corn and children. I told
him that I would feel very much at home—with corn and children. That's what I remember most about my first visit to Walstonburg. I'm sure they hadn't started construction yet.[12]

Schafer, from the rural farming area of southern Illinois, feels that her
line about feeling at home with growing corn and children was what sold
the board on her as a candidate for the Walstonburg clinic.

Schafer came to North Carolina in September 1972. Prepared as a
pediatric nurse practitioner initially, she came to Chapel Hill first to complete the adult health portion of the Nurse Practitioner Program. Schafer
would also accompany Bernstein or Pergrin to Walstonburg, meeting with
the board, interviewing the support staff, providing input on the clinic

building plans, and, most importantly, meeting with Dr. Beddingfield, who would be her backup physician. After Donna finished the adult portion of the curriculum and passed the final exam, covering adults and children, she was "certified by exam" as a graduate of the UNC-CH Family Nurse Practitioner Program. On March 10, 1973, the Walstonburg clinic opened, with Donna Schafer its first nurse practitioner.

Hot Springs Community Health Center

The Hot Springs clinic opened on May 1, 1971—with a hope and a prayer and $500, thanks to the activism and persistence of Linda Mashburn.[13] She, a public health nurse, and a few community volunteers ran the clinic until Mashburn was able to recruit a nurse practitioner. Mashburn was also running into a few problems with local physicians and pharmacists. She had previously met Don Madison at a Department of Health, Education, and Welfare conference in DC. Madison was now at UNC-CH, and she contacted him for advice and help. In July, Madison went to Hot Springs, in Madison County, and he brought along Bernstein, Sheps, and Julia Watkins from the FNP Program.

At that time Mashburn learned about the training program in Chapel Hill and how it might be useful to her plans for Hot Springs. About a year later, with funding from the Z. Smith Reynolds Foundation and the Appalachian Regional Commission, Mashburn was able to recruit Linda Tull, an adult nurse practitioner from Boston. Tull, like Schafer before her, spent some months in Chapel Hill for pediatric training and completion of final exams; Tull was then certified by the UNC program as a family nurse practitioner. In 1972, two additional nurses sponsored by the Hot Springs clinic enrolled in the FNP Program.

However, the clinic in Hot Springs had its growing pains and challenges —like all the other early clinics. Her contacts in Chapel Hill, including

Don Madison, helped her and the community leaders get through opposition from the local medical societies and area pharmacists. This help came from two new innovative programs under development at UNC.

COINCIDENTAL AND SYNCHRONOUS INNOVATIONS

During the late sixties and early to mid-seventies, a readiness to innovate, an eagerness to respond to the needs for health services and education in the state, and a commitment to interdisciplinary collaboration characterized many new developments in the Health Affairs Division at UNC. This spirit of activism—to a degree unusual for university faculty—is recalled with fondness by those involved at the time.

The first innovation was the Family Nurse Practitioner Program—a program of the School of Nursing but with sponsorship from the School of Medicine and the School of Public Health, with considerable involvement of faculty from the School of Medicine. Two other innovative and well-known programs developed at UNC around the same time, and many of the same individuals were involved in each of them. Any discussion of the NP movement in North Carolina must include reference to the North Carolina Area Health Education Centers and the North Carolina Rural Health Program—as they turned out to be synergistic and complementary programs to one another.

The North Carolina Area Health Education Centers (AHEC)

When Glenn Wilson came to UNC to consult with those involved in starting the NP Program, the Prospect Hill clinic, and the UNC–OCCHS partnership, he had no idea he would eventually end up permanently at UNC. Shortly after, he joined the UNC faculty as the director of the division of education and research in community care—the division where most of the physicians interested in primary care services affiliated. Wilson wrote a grant to help the OCCHS Program get started.

When the medical school decided to double its class size, they did not have the capacity to provide clinical experiences for all the additional students. So Wilson, now associate dean for community health services, developed affiliations with hospitals across the state for medical student clinical experiences and received funds from the state legislature for these outreach efforts.[14]

In the summer of 1972, Wilson unexpectedly received a call from Congressman Charles L. Vanik of Ohio, where Wilson was before coming to UNC. According to Wilson,

Vanik told me of a Health Manpower Bill that included money for off-campus training. Vanik said, write a grant; otherwise, $2.5 million will revert to the federal coffers. The Health Manpower Bill did not include the term "AHEC," only off-campus training. However, a recent Carnegie report had used the term "AHEC," and thus, the UNC proposal described a statewide AHEC system.... Faye Pickard, Glenn Pickard, John Payne, Gene Mayer, and Shirley O'Keefe [Glenn's secretary] joined Wilson in writing the proposal that initiated the North Carolina AHEC Program.[15]

Faye Pickard describes the grant-writing scene.

We'd [Faye and Glenn Pickard] go to the beach. We would tape a proposal, and we'd put the tapes on the airplane—the little airplane would land at Ocean Isle. We would send tapes back to Chapel Hill. The tapes would come back the next day, typed out, rough draft, and we would send more tapes back. We would work on the rough drafts, send it back, and in three or four days, we would come home, and the thing would be typed by the time we got here. Then we would "walk it through" administration to get it to Audrey [Booth, School of Nursing acting dean in the summer] in time—with people having read rough drafts as they came out of the typewriter. It was absolutely wild.[16]

The grant was completed and submitted in time, and an $8.5 million federal contract was awarded to the medical school to develop a state-wide AHEC program. The state also allocated $2.6 million to support phase one of program development. Wilson became the first director of the North Carolina AHEC Program.

The program's stated goal was to develop centers across the state to improve the quantity, quality, and distribution of health care professionals. With seven centers strategically located across the state, each center would provide training and continuing education opportunities for all the health professions—serving as magnets to attract professionals to rural and underserved areas. Three AHEC centers established initially included Charlotte Memorial Hospital, New Hanover Memorial Hospital, and a coalition of hospitals that became the Area L AHEC.[17] The Area L AHEC, and the Mountain AHEC, which developed later, became essential links to further expansion of the NP Program.

The Rural Health Program

Jim Bernstein continued to work with the Walstonburg community to develop its clinic. Because the first local Walstonburg nurse practitioner moved away, Bernstein was instrumental in connecting Donna Schafer to the community. But he felt Walstonburg needed further development. Bernstein's interest was in community development, and he wanted to test a different approach to help rural communities secure health services. Bernstein's focus was on providing technical and business assistance to help communities build, own, and operate their clinics. He often discussed his ideas and thinking with Sheps. Sheps had opportunities to talk with legislators occasionally, and because Bernstein was working with Sheps during his fellowship years, Sheps told legislators about the kinds of things Bernstein was doing.[18]

State legislators were very interested in the measures the medical and nursing schools were taking to alleviate the state's rural health problem. James Holshouser, elected governor of North Carolina in 1972—the first Republican governor in the twentieth century and since Reconstruction—served his first term in the North Carolina House of Representatives in 1963–65. He was a native of rural Watauga County in western North Carolina. During his first term, he experienced firsthand the day-to-day developments of legislative study committees, and from them he learned how complex health care issues were. He had also served in the House in 1969 during the study of the shortage of physicians in rural areas. Thus, his immersion in many political tugs of war sensitized Holshouser to the realities of medical and state politics. It also readied him for backing successful health care legislation when he was elected governor in 1972.

Shortly after Holshouser was elected governor, he called Vice Chancellor of Health Affairs Sheps, who relates his conversation with the governor.

[Holshouser] said, "I want to come to talk with you about this rural stuff. I think it is important." He had tremendous intelligence—really understanding.... I said to him, look, it's only two programs, but we're confident this will work, and this will work in many places. Then we got a hold of Bill [William] Friday [president of the UNC University System], and Bill was involved, and so on. Holshouser said, "Well, I'd like to propose this and develop a plan and a budget." So, we did. The budget provided for the Office of Rural Health Services, and funding, on a matching basis, for facilities, and subsidization at a limited level for three years....

He started by saying that he wanted the university to run it. I said
no, no, I don't think we should. It should be a state function.[19]

[Glenn] Wilson also discussed the question about where the Office
of Rural Health should be housed—in the university or in state government. While the new budget was under development for the AHEC
Program, Holshouser added funding for the Rural Health Program. He
called a special session of the legislature to address these programs. As
Wilson recalled,

> Holshouser went on to publicly endorse nurse practitioners...
> because he began to hear from the constituents who were receiv-
> ing services, including Hot Springs, Walstonburg, and around here
> [Prospect Hill]. It appealed to him as a way to do things.... He
> originally proposed that AHEC, which had been developed, and
> the Office of Rural Health, be all in one program.... [M]y recollec-
> tion is quite clear. I told the president [of the university] that we did
> not want the Office of Rural Health, that the university should not
> do this. Universities didn't do those things very well.[20]

The Rural Health Program was funded by the legislature, as were the
AHEC Program and the NP Program. Holshouser was true to his word.
"Jim [Bernstein] was technically placed in the North Carolina Department
of Human Resources, but [Jim] literally worked for the governor directly.
He [Gov. Holshouser] kept all the politicians and bureaucracy at bay."[21]

A remarkable part of these developments is that all this transpired
before the legal status of nurse practitioners had been addressed. But at
this stage, nurse practitioners had some very prominent advocates. As
Sheps told key legislators at a dinner hosted by the governor before a
"called" joint session of the House and Senate,

Well, during the presentation after dinner, I said, now, I want you to understand, I'm not talking about something [nurse practitioners] that's a poor substitute. I'm talking about something that's not only as good, but I think it's better—not only because it's permanent, but because I think it will do things that the average doctor doesn't do.[22]

Wilson gave a similar endorsement:

It was sold to the governor and others as a way to deal with North Carolina's problems. At least I said to the governor and Lieutenant Governor Hunt, very clearly, we are going to set out to train people for whom the second order of priority, if any priority at all, will be upward mobility. We are deliberately going to train people who will be in North Carolina to take care of North Carolina's problems. Any registered nurse is qualified. We are not into the credentials business; we are not going to get into those kinds of controversies.[23]

Governor Holshouser himself provided a similar account:

I had seen sometime [in] the last two or three weeks before the election in 1972 an article on the pilot program, I think it was Walstonburg—it could have been Hot Springs—and just thought to myself, hmm, after the election, if things go right, that's something we ought to look into. I stopped by to see Bill Friday [president of the University of North Carolina System] sometime.... I told him I would like to talk to him some time or another about this idea and have him bring in the people who had been involved in that operation. So early on in the administration, probably in

January—it may have been February, but I think it was January—
we had a dinner at the mansion. [President Friday] brought over
Cecil Sheps and some other people from the university. I guess
Chris Fordham was probably there—it was probably eight or ten
people, to talk about the program that had been developed under
the federal grant. We talked about the AHECs [Area Health Education Centers] at the same time, and that was a logical component if you were going to try to put together a composite program,
and we talked about how you'd go about starting.[24]

Governor Holshouser reflected on the successes of the Rural Health
and Nurse Practitioner Programs:

It's been encouraging as a project to see something that didn't
require a huge infusion of state or federal funds, because in most
cases the programs are self-supporting after about three years, and
a good bit of the seed money is raised at the local level, so it really
is a community project in the financial sense. Of course, the key to
it all is the practitioner. You've got to have the community support
and people with some leadership ability who can put together a
fundraising drive and get a site selected, this sort of thing. Then
you've got to have a nurse practitioner, and it was amazing to me
that in so many cases, you had nurses from the community who
were available to go to school about it.[25]

From 1972 through 1978, the development of the Nurse Practitioner,
AHEC, and Rural Health Programs were, in many ways, symbiotic. They
grew up, side-by-side, like neighbor kids. They helped each other out.
They did not compete. In some ways, they were dependent on each other
initially. Each helped the other in their achievements. When they finally

grew up, each, in their own right and on their own, were successes. Many of the same people were involved in or helped out all of the programs as they developed. A loosely coupled network was evolving. At its hub was the FNP Policy Board.

At this point, curricular matters and admissions were handled by program faculty. But with the development of the sister programs (AHEC and Rural Health) and the growing number of nurse practitioner practice sites across the state, there was a need for key leaders to come together to develop political strategies and oversee the rapid escalation of what was becoming a statewide movement. Many of those appointed to the initial FNP Policy Board, usually just known as the Policy Board, had worked together informally to develop plans and strategies. But now it was becoming more important that all the leaders were on the same page.

In theory, the Policy Board was advisory to the dean of the School of Nursing. But the Policy Board did not operate on hierarchical principles. They had always interacted collegially and informally, and there was no reason to change that. But there was a need to formalize representation on the Policy Board. In addition to Lucy Conant, dean of nursing, there was a representative of the dean of medicine—initially Glenn Wilson and then Eugene Mayer in 1973—and a representative of the dean of the School of Public Health—initially Marie McIntyre and then Julia Watkins in 1972. Audrey Booth returned to the School of Nursing full-time and became a member of the Policy Board. And when the Rural Health Program began, Jim Bernstein also joined the Policy Board. Others were invited to specific meetings depending on the topic or issue being addressed.

While the Policy Board was evolving and developing strategies that would support the success of all of the complementary programs working to solve the state's rural health care crisis, the Chapel Hill FNP Program admitted another nineteen students from all parts of the state. Between the third class of students at Chapel Hill and the six AHEC students in

1973–74, another twenty-five nurse practitioners were prepared for practice in in all regions of North Carolina. By the end of 1974, ten Rural Health Program community sites were in some phase of development.

The next chapters will discuss the NP movement's expanding educational programs, including a trial satellite program and consortium development, legal and professional issues, and the dedicated network that managed and maneuvered through these issues.

CHAPTER EIGHT

The New Order Expands:
NP Movement Goes Statewide

Note to Reader: Throughout this chapter, in various sections, I switch to first person point of view because I am the major and often sole informant of the narrative.

Despite proximity to UNC, counties surrounding the medical center in Chapel Hill, namely Orange and Chatham, were underserved, lacking a source of primary care. When the medical school was authorized to expand in the early 1950s, the school and hospital were given a mandate to develop as a referral-only medical center. The mandate was the result of physicians in the state raising concern about their own practices, fearing UNC would take their private patients as their own. The specialty-oriented UNC physicians did not see this as an issue; they wanted to see patients with complicated biological problems and had no interest in providing day-to-day ongoing care—what we know today as primary care.

Consequently, as if a wall surrounded the medical center, local citizens were left out and without an ongoing source of care. This system deficit prompted Jim Bryan to initiate the continuing care clinic. In essence, he opened the door of the medical center to locals seeking a source of continuing care. When Pickard returned to UNC and joined Bryan in the continuing care clinic, they both realized that nurses could do much more than the current system allowed, so they began teaching nurses expanded skills. These nurses provided much-needed continuing care not only in the clinic, but also "out in the community and in patient's homes." As noted previously, these forces and changes ultimately led to the formalization of the Family Nurse Practitioner Program.

Six of the seven graduates of the first class of the Family Nurse Practitioner Program at UNC were destined to serve clinics in the counties immediately surrounding the UNC Medical Center. In two years, forty-two nurse practitioners practiced in clinics and doctor's offices across the state. There continued to be a demand for primary care services and a demand from nurses, and physicians, for nurse practitioner training, even though the nurse practitioner role was still viewed with suspicion by many other nurses and doctors.

In 1973, to meet these demands, the FNP Program Policy Board made two consequential decisions. One decision was to admit two classes per year. With the Rural Health Program fully operational, helping communities develop their own local system of health care services, the program leadership needed assurances that UNC could provide the number of nurse practitioners needed for the new rural health clinics. The FNP Policy Board assured the Rural Health Program of at least six to eight student placements in each class for the next few years. So, in 1973, the program admitted students in September and in March/April. As a result, the yearly nurse practitioner graduation rate doubled, as did the need for additional faculty.

Judy Watkins, now the nursing codirector of the program, Conant, and Pickard all recognized the importance of a mix of nurse practitioners and physicians teaching students, reflecting their underlying belief in the collegial nature of the nurse practitioner–physician relationship and the blending of different levels and kinds of expertise. Clara Milko, a pediatric nurse practitioner, joined the faculty, and Margaret Wilkman divided her time between clinical practice at Prospect Hill and at the School of Nursing.

Carolyn Williams had also joined the FNP faculty earlier in 1971, but her primary responsibilities were as coprincipal investigator for the PRIMEX grant. The PRIMEX grant was a demonstration project, including a significant evaluation component. Conant felt she needed to have a nurse researcher in charge of the evaluation requirements of the grant. Consequently, Williams was not involved in teaching nurse practitioner students; instead, she worked full-time administering the grant. Over time, however, she hired additional faculty for the grant, including a nurse practitioner from the Rochester NP Program and a recent master's graduate from Yale University, which added to the rich mix of program faculty. The blending of nurse practitioners and physicians as faculty reflected the increasing maturing of the nurse practitioner movement.

The second consequential decision of the Policy Board was to initiate a satellite FNP program in the fall of 1973 in the Area L AHEC. Satellite programs would also help meet the burgeoning demand for nurse practitioners and community-based services.

A SATELLITE NP PROGRAM TRIAL

The notion of developing satellite programs in the state was not a new one. From the beginning of the NP Program, concern about the difficulties involved in getting nurses to come to Chapel Hill for six months had been raised. Most were family-bound to their hometowns. Furthermore, as Faye Pickard recalls,

[W]e were also concerned that we had inadvertently ended up recruiting students who came here for six months, but instead of going back to their communities, they ended up at Orange–

Chatham. We felt the need to carry forward our basic belief that it was best to educate people as close to their home as possible. We talked about the day when we could have satellite programs out in the state from the very beginning.... Wilmington was to be the site of our first satellite program because of the interest there [and] because of a school of nursing there.[1]

When the Pickards, Wilson, and others wrote the first AHEC proposal, a satellite program was planned for Wilmington AHEC—under the assumption that the Wilmington AHEC would be the first to have the desire and capacity to offer such a program. However, Wilmington was not ready. But Dr. Lawrence (Larry) Cutchin in the Area L AHEC at Tarboro, North Carolina, was.

Larry Cutchin followed Glenn Pickard as chief resident in medicine. As young physicians, they advocated for primary care, and wanted it to have significant visibility in the medical school. But they knew that was a long shot. They concluded that they needed a new model and had many conversations about how to advance the concept of nurse practitioners across the state and beyond. Since they both had worked with nurses who were experienced in dealing with everyday common health problems, they knew that nurses responded to the needs of people, and that people who knew them as nurses trusted them. They also knew that nurses helped many in their communities, even if not socially or institutionally authorized to do so. Consequently, Pickard and Cutchin advocated for more education and increased recognition for nurses.

Cutchin finished his residency and moved back to Tarboro, North Carolina, to join a group practice affiliated with a local hospital. The Tarboro Hospital, part of a coalition of hospitals that had joined to form a regional AHEC, became the primary hub of the Area L AHEC, with Cutchin as its director. When the Wilmington AHEC option for a satellite NP program faltered, Pickard put on his thinking cap, just about the time I returned to Chapel Hill to defend my thesis in March 1973.

During my two years as a graduate student, I had talked with Glenn Pickard weekly—and learned, vicariously, about every developmental, curricular, and political struggle faced by the NP advocates during the first two years of the program. We became good friends and shared the same desire to "make things better" and to take on a cause no matter the obstacles. Our reconnection in March got Glenn rethinking the satellite program option.

In early spring 1973, I returned home to Wisconsin, my thesis defense successful, with a graduate degree in hand. During the course of my graduate studies, I had learned about a new way of doing and thinking about nursing practice. I did not know where I would land or what I would try next but knew it would be different and would derive from what I had learned and experienced at UNC. One month later during one of the most severe Milwaukee snowstorms in years—six feet of snow within a few hours, a five-hour drive home from work in what was usually a twenty-minute ride—I received a phone call from Glenn. That phone call changed my life plan.

It wasn't a long conversation, but Glenn Pickard had called with what he described as a "great opportunity." My recollection of the phone call was that, simply put, Glenn's idea was for me to come back to North Carolina to start the first satellite FNP program in the AHEC located in Tarboro. Glenn described Tarboro as an affluent southern town in the eastern part of the state. As a graduate student, I knew Chapel Hill. I had traveled to the coast and to the mountains of North Carolina—but nowhere in between. I had no idea where Tarboro was. Glenn also described Larry (Cutchin) and Larry's interest in and support for nurse practitioners.

Denied my chance to become a nurse practitioner a year ago while a graduate student, I was not going to pass up another. I told Glenn I would seriously consider the "opportunity"—IF I could also take the program as a student while I planned and directed the program, thereby earning a certificate as a family nurse practitioner.

Glenn, who can sell just about anything, sang the praises of this southern town and a great opportunity for a northerner who had just survived shoveling tons of snow! A couple of weeks later, I was on a plane to Chapel Hill to meet with Glenn, Larry Cutchin, and Audrey Booth, now director of statewide AHEC nursing activities. For me, it was a done deal. In June, I moved to North Carolina without having laid eyes on Tarboro. I started organizing the curriculum and faculty and admitted six students, including myself, to the first satellite FNP program in North Carolina.

The satellite program was an "experiment," another pilot program. Would it work? Would it be successful if conducted quite a distance from a medical center where there were experienced teaching faculty? Would practicing physicians in the area be willing to teach classes? Would there be sufficient and diverse clinical experiences in the area for student learning experiences? Would the practicing physicians available in the area be ready and have the know-how to guide the students' clinical skills? Most importantly, after the preceptorship, would students pass the final exam given to all FNP students at Chapel Hill? These questions would be tested in the Area L satellite pilot program.

Because of my experience in curriculum development, I began to reorganize the FNP curriculum, adding more detail to the curricular outline. I discussed various classroom and clinical teaching needs with physicians at the Tarboro clinic—because the clinic was only five minutes away from the FNP classroom. They were willing, but they were not sure how they would accommodate six nurse practitioner students in their small clinic, particularly when medical students came from Chapel Hill for a "rural" experience.

Getting the number and type of clinical experiences needed for the six students was tight. I also realized that I needed to bring in faculty from

UNC to teach certain classroom topics, which turned out to be useful because students were then exposed to nurses and physicians who had worked with nurse practitioners. As the six-month classroom and clinical teaching portion of the program was coming to a close, I did not question the need for satellite FNP programs across the state. To me, the question was not if, but rather how, where, and with what resources.

In the spring, while the students were in their preceptorships, Pickard, Booth, Cutchin, and I, plus other AHEC staff, considered the ongoing feasibility of a satellite program through a rural AHEC such as the Area L AHEC. I had concluded that the primary difficulty was faculty. Local physicians from the area were willing but could not take time from busy practices to teach classes. Further, they did not have experience in classroom teaching. Nor did they have the time and inclination to provide clinical experiences and supervision. What was needed by NP students was different than the medical teaching model used in medical schools, which is what most of the local physicians knew. I also had a sense that a new and developing AHEC was not yet ready to take on a year-long program of study.

I had been aware there was a School of Nursing in Greenville, North Carolina, twenty-eight miles away. I didn't know much about the school, just that there was one—at East Carolina University (ECU). Up to now, I had spent only six months in eastern North Carolina. Immersed in setting up and running the FNP Program, I knew very little, if anything, about the professional–political issues there. But Booth and Pickard gave me a crash course in the medical–professional–political dynamics of eastern North Carolina. Booth was acutely aware that other nursing schools in the state were sensitive to and cautious about overreach on the part of the Chapel Hill School of Nursing. Thus, any overture to ECU's nursing school had to be approached delicately, with a clear sense of collaboration and partnership.

Pickard felt that the Board of Medical Examiners and the Medical Society would require certain assurances about any new programs that might develop in the eastern and western parts of the state. These groups implicitly agreed not to interfere with or oppose the UNC program because they were informed about and acknowledged the program's quality and its faculty and curriculum. Pickard felt a need to say that other programs were similar—without imposing UNC's curriculum on partner programs, a sensitive path to navigate. Compounding matters was everyone's desire not to get the FNP Program expansion goals embroiled in the controversy about a new medical school at ECU.

Eastern AHEC, in Greenville and affiliated with ECU, was just getting organized in early 1974. Each regional AHEC would have a director of nursing programs, and Terri Lawler was the first such director for Eastern AHEC. According to Evelyn Perry, dean of the ECU School of Nursing, she and Ed Monroe, the first director of Eastern AHEC, had many conversations about how to get support from the AHEC for the Nurse Practitioner Program. Monroe felt it unwise to bring this issue before the physician-dominated AHEC board. Instead, he assured her that there would be funding "pretty well hidden" in the budget for the program.[2]

There would not be overt public support from the new Eastern AHEC, but Perry and Lawler attribute much support for nurse practitioners to Ed Beddingfield, Lawrence Cutchin, and Jim Bernstein; they helped calm opposition to NPs. Soon Perry was able to say that public health departments were asking for nurse practitioners, and Bernstein needed them for rural health clinics in the east. Perry could then point to demand.

Perry and Lawler were aware of the program in Tarboro, and felt it was a Chapel Hill–Cutchin thing, a satellite program to prepare NPs for the Tarboro clinic. Cutchin, although philosophically in agreement with Chapel Hill, resisted their influence and meddling in his affairs. Thus, he was in support of the program moving to ECU. Further, Lucy Conant was not territorial about any regional nurse practitioner program. Perry recalled a meeting with Conant in which Conant endorsed the idea of a nurse practitioner program in the east. She further assuaged Perry's fear of dominance by Chapel Hill, recalling that Conant never felt there were any territorial rights. With that assurance, Perry readied the ECU School of Nursing for a nurse practitioner program. She sought and was awarded federal funds in 1975.[3]

Conant had not been involved directly with the Tarboro arrangement. With the program underway, she allowed Pickard and Booth to be the front persons as needed. Perry recalled, "It was a Glenn Pickard, via Larry Cutchin, via Cindy, via Booth, via the Area L AHEC arrangement."[4] In many ways, that is how things happened in the early nurse practitioner days. You knew the end goal—or at least Pickard did—and when an opportunity came, he or we grabbed it. He had many "unofficial" conversations with Cutchin and Perry. And likely, Pickard discussed these issues in Policy Board meetings and had many background conversations with all those involved in considering the ECU program so that everyone was on the same page when the formal meetings occurred.

A STATE TASK FORCE, THE CONSORTIUM'S BEGINNINGS

Perry was getting increasing pressure from Jim Bernstein to develop a nurse practitioner program, who needed NPs for rural clinics in the east; from Ed Travathen, director of the Greenville Health Department; and from a few local physicians. She knew this was the way to go but was not getting much financial support from the new Eastern AHEC, and the School of Nursing did not have the funds to start such an endeavor without additional support.

Booth had met with Perry on many occasions related to the new Eastern AHEC—and gently introduced the idea of a possible NP program at ECU. Pickard went to Greenville to meet with Perry, Lawler, and others at ECU and in the Greenville area. One meeting gave Perry and Lawler some assurance that UNC wanted to be helpful.

In late September 1974, Booth and I met with Perry—the first time Perry and I had met. This meeting carried some import. I had returned to Chapel Hill, joining the faculty of the FNP Program as associate director for outreach programs, which later was retitled AHEC liaison for nurse practitioner programs—a soon-to-be created position funded by Central AHEC. However, Perry would have no way of knowing, never having met me, that my approach to most efforts was collaborative. But as far as Perry knew, I was coming from Chapel Hill. I needed to tread lightly and certainly not as a "know-it-all," giving Perry time to make her own assessment of my capability, trustworthiness, and objectives.

I remember that meeting quite well, as I felt the weight of developing a successful relationship with the dean of a sister nursing school. Our plans to expand nurse practitioner programs in the state were dependent on mutually respectful relationships. You know quickly when you are meeting someone like-minded. That was a mutual takeaway. Perry, Booth, and I agreed to call a joint meeting of our faculties in Greenville in October (1974), which would include Booth, Pickard, Watkins, and me from UNC-CH, and Lawler, Penry,[5] and Perry from ECU. We all met at the Greenville Country Club for lunch—the first time anything about an NP program at ECU was formally discussed. Lawler described the meeting:

> I remember approaching it very tentatively and thinking we're going to be treated like upstarts and maybe even second-class citizenry. The physicians are going to monopolize the conversation, and they're going to go through the old discussion of control and all that jazz. My perception was that Evelyn started. I don't remember what she said…. She must have set such a positive tone and a positive stage that we never had to go through whether this would be a good thing.[6]

Perry added, "It was: How can we help you get it started?" Lawler amplified:

How can we help? Because I can remember Glenn Pickard and I talking, and we all sat in a circle. It was either a round table or we'd pulled the chairs in a circle because I remember sitting in a circle. I remember Glenn and I were opposite each other, and all of a sudden, from political issues and everything else, we got into "How are we going to fix the curriculum?" That's right. Glenn said, "I've always wanted to use modules, but I've never been able to convince anybody." There was this big bridge that suddenly was spanned, and it wasn't WE are going to do it, but HOW are we going to do it?[7]

In a follow-up meeting that afternoon with Perry and Booth, I was charged with writing a memorandum of agreement between the two schools—ECU and UNC. Now words would be on paper, and they had to be thoughtfully written.

I took a long time to write that memo. It was more than a simple follow-up reminder of a next meeting. It was a political statement that would signal a new era and relationship between the two schools of nursing. It had to convey that we were on equal footing in this endeavor, that we were committed to a common goal, and that we would work together toward this end. It was a short, four-sentence statement of understanding, which referenced a second meeting in December 1974. The memo stated, quite simply:

A general agreement was reached that UNC-CH and ECU work together and collaborate in making their respective FNP programs as similar as possible. As a result of this agreement, the above-named people will meet as a task force on December 8th and 9th to discuss the nature and extent of this collaborative effort. In preparation for this retreat, ECU and UNC will exchange proposals and curricular materials by November 8th. Evelyn Perry and Cindy Freund will set the agenda, and Audrey Booth and Cindy Freund will make the meeting arrangements.[8]

The memorandum of agreement was accepted by all parties and set the stage for the upcoming retreat.

While Perry agreed to continue discussions about an NP program in the east and to collaborate with UNC-CH, at ECU, like Conant a few years before, Perry also had to contend with a faculty that was not in full support of nurse practitioners. According to Lawler,

> Our [ECU] faculty, I think, was very suspicious of [Allison Armstrong[9]] as a nurse practitioner. They didn't understand what a nurse practitioner was. They thought that she was a junior doctor who was selling out nursing. She was never well received by our faculty, though she was a neat gal and very, very skilled…. Allison built bridges much more readily with the physicians—the pediatricians— who really did accept her and liked her, valuing her skills; the other physicians tolerated her. [She built bridges with physicians] much more easily than she did with nursing. I think she had a terrible case of reality shock when she tried to become integrated into our faculty. I think she never really was able, first of all, to articulate her role successfully, and I think they treated her very badly as a result.[10]

Perry added: "[T]here was an attitude prevalent in nursing then. We haven't conquered it yet, [but the prevalent attitude was] that nurses who go into the Nurse Practitioner Program are deserting nursing and that all they are doing is the low-paid stuff that physicians don't want to do."[11] Like Conant before her, Perry moved forward with a nurse practitioner program without the majority of her faculty's support. It was the only way to move forward in those days, the early '70s.

Soon Perry had hired other faculty, namely Judy Garrison, Phyllis Nichols, Lona Ratcliffe, and Nancy Stamey. UNC also recruited an additional nurse practitioner to the faculty. Ruth Ouimette, an FNP graduate of the Bates–Lynaugh Pilot Program at the University of Rochester (New York), and a recent graduate of Yale University's master's program came to work with Williams on the PRIMEX grant and with the FNP Program faculty. In addition, she was the first nurse practitioner to hold a graduate faculty appointment in the School of Nursing—a real coup, allowing her to work with graduate students.

The group named itself the "Statewide Task Force of Family Nurse Practitioner Programs." The December retreat, at the beach at Nags Head, provided everyone time to discuss issues and get to know each other. They continued to meet, in January in Chapel Hill and in May in Greenville, and then they planned another retreat, a three-day retreat at the beach in Morehead City. By May, Perry had managed to hire Donna Schafer, from the Walstonburg clinic, as the FNP Program director— and ECU set a starting date, October 6, 1975, for its first class.

Again, the retreat provided the faculty an ideal way to get to know each other, to have small working-group time, and to have the group take ownership of this partnership. Various groups had worked by phone in the interim, preparing and sharing material. Everyone involved, when reflecting on these retreats, described them as extremely productive— and fun! And they were proud of their collaboration, colleagueship, and developing friendships.

A STATEWIDE NURSE PRACTITIONER CONSORTIUM

By fall 1975, and only one year later, more faculty were recruited to the effort, both at ECU and UNC, and additional physicians joined: Larry

Cutchin and Jim Jones from ECU, and Frank Loda from UNC. By September 1975, the Task Force expanded in another way, this time including faculty from a program starting in the western part of the state, a program sponsored by the Mountain AHEC (MAHEC)—Hettie Garland and Katherine (Kit) Nuckols.

I had met Hettie Garland at the ANA convention in 1974. Our shared memory is sitting in a Kansas City bar with an entourage of North Carolina nurse practitioners. We asked the pianist to play "Carolina in the Morning"—to which all rose in spirited voice to sing along. That was Hettie's and my first meeting, well-remembered, though we did not know whether a second encounter would ever occur. The second meeting took place in Glenn Pickard's office at UNC, where he and I were meeting—likely talking about troubles in the western part of the state.

In walked Garland. Glenn jumped up, gave her a hearty hug—as he always does—and proceeded to introduce Hettie to me. I then sprang up to hug Garland, joyful to reconnect—while Glenn watched on, wondering, "How do these two know each other?" Garland happened to be in Chapel Hill with her physician–husband, who was inquiring about a family practice residency in the planning throes by Mountain AHEC. He was interviewing for a position there.

Pickard and I gave each other the "eye," the "you-know-what-I'm-thinking" look. Then we both told Garland about the under-the-cover plan for a nurse practitioner program at Mountain AHEC (MAHEC). The only nursing school in the western part of the state, Western Carolina University (WCU), was new and struggling, without faculty or resources to offer a nurse practitioner program—nor did they want to. According to Katherine "Kit" Nuckolls, the nursing affairs MAHEC director, "The new dean at Western Carolina came from Martha Rogers's program,[12] so she was not in favor of nurse practitioners, nor interested. So, there was no real interest or support from that faculty at that time."[13] Consequently, the Mountain AHEC was the best possible option for an FNP program in the west, so Pickard and I gave this growing idea the best pitch possible. When all was said and done, all three of us were excited about the possibility of starting a nurse practitioner program at the Mountain AHEC in the western part of the state.

Of course, there were a few "I"s to dot and "T"s to cross—such as convincing the director of MAHEC, Henry Uhl, that it was time to start a nurse practitioner program. Even if not prepared, he was ready, so it was not difficult to get him on board. But it was even more important to convince the newly hired MAHEC director of nursing affairs, Nuckolls, that Hettie Garland was the person to lead the program. Nuckolls, Booth, and Conant had always hoped WCU would offer the program— but they agreed that MAHEC should start the program with me as a ready consultant to Garland.

In January 1975, Garland returned for an interview with Nuckolls and me. As Garland remembers the day,

I went back in January and met with you [referring to me] and Kit. That was my first interview with Kit. You and Kit were essentially spending the day together, sitting in her office, developing that original equipment list. In fact, I think I still have that list. [Kit] was coming back and forth [from Yale] as a consultant even then and working periodically there [in Asheville]. We [all] had a conversation with Henry at the end of the day, because Kit's primary concern was my not having a master's degree. But at the end of the day, she felt comfortable. Henry offered me the job and said that what he was getting was kind of a husband-and-wife team.... They were killing two birds with one stone in terms of Don's [Hettie's husband] being full-time, the only full-time family medicine faculty member with the residency program, and the affiliation that I had with UNC. I think that naturally led to the position. I didn't come back until April, when we met again, and then I got started in July. Lydia [a staff member at MAHEC] had already gathered about ten to fifteen applications for the program.[14]

Garland had five months to pull things together as the program start date was October 1975. Fortunately, by that time, UNC and ECU had developed a standard curriculum with accompanying program materials. Garland's initial priorities were selecting students and identifying teachers and clinical preceptors. She recalls that Harry Summerlin, a physician with MAHEC,

was a big facilitator in that, because he helped me pick out physicians, ones he knew, who he thought were good teachers, and who he thought would relate to the nurse practitioner concept.[15]

Garland had no problem recruiting students. The plan had been to admit only six students to the first MAHEC class—but Uhl, MAHEC's director, had made prior commitments. Consequently, the first MAHEC class started with ten students—and fortunately, there was enough stipend money from MAHEC to support ten students.

Most of the students in the first class were from the Asheville area, and they were crucial in selling the nurse practitioner role to the community. One month before starting the program in MAHEC, Garland joined the Statewide Task Force—renamed the "North Carolina Consortium of Nurse Practitioner Programs." Nuckolls also joined the Statewide Task Force. She helped Garland with the initial program start-up work and then felt confident in Garland's ability to manage it. And, even more, she was confident in Garland's ability to manage all the politics associated with the nurse practitioner movement. As director of nursing programs for MAHEC, her participation in the consortium was appropriate; she joined her counterpart from the EAHEC. There were now, in 1975, nurse practitioner programs in all three areas of the state, representative of its natural divisions: the west, central Piedmont, and eastern parts of North Carolina, from the mountains to the sea.

DIFFUSION AND MATURING OF THE MOVEMENT

The North Carolina Consortium of Nurse Practitioner Programs did more than achieve its original intention to ensure consistency among program curricula and adherence to agreed-upon objectives and outcomes. The consortium members, collaboratively, and in alliance, endorsed a definition of a "family nurse practitioner." They also worked side by side to develop standardized exams. And they developed a standard curriculum. Laurel Copp[16] recalled Nuckolls's description of the "common curriculum": "Remember Kit's term, 'controlled diversity'? We wanted to do something similar, but we didn't want cookie-cutter programs all across the state. I think we were able to achieve that."[17] All of this is difficult to do within one faculty in one school. Special interests, "pet" theories, and emphases can be debated with vigor. But this was not characteristic of the interaction among and work of the consortium members. Of course, there were differing opinions. These were aired and listened to respectfully, with compromise leading to the eventual conclusion. The regulatory and professional bodies of both medicine and nursing in the state were assured that in North Carolina, "a nurse practitioner was a nurse practitioner." North Carolina could avoid degree muddle in relation to nurse practitioners prepared in the state.

By 1975, three programs, not just one, were preparing nurse practitioners for the state. The two new programs at ECU and MAHEC started with small class sizes, but they quickly expanded their enrollments to keep up with demand. In 1975, before the start of the two new programs, over one hundred nurse practitioners had graduated from the UNC program. By 1978, over three hundred nurse practitioners from all three programs were in practice in North Carolina, a threefold increase.[18]

The consortium accomplished more than increasing the supply of nurse practitioners and assuring consistency among its NP programs. Each program alone had only a few medical and nursing faculty to exchange ideas about program issues and future directions. In the consortium arena, in contrast, there were considerably more faculty and thus more ideas to consider. The consortium provided fertile ground to nourish and flesh out new ideas, new approaches—and that is what happened. Equally important, consortium members included doctors and nurses. Each wanted the other's input and involvement. Neither dominated the other. The relationship among nurse and physician faculty and those with and without titled positions mirrored the relationship the early founders of the Nurse Practitioner Program wanted to engender between nurse practitioners and physicians—colleagueship and learning from the other's expertise.

Early on, the consortium decided to organize curricular guidelines in modules, such as adult health, child health, maternal and women's health, geriatric health, and a common core. All of these modules combined formed the nexus for a family nurse practitioner curriculum. The modules also allowed each program to prepare nurse practitioners to focus on specific population groups—and some of them did so. For example, in the eastern part of the state, there were more requests from local and county health departments for pediatric nurse practitioners (PNPs) and maternal and women's health practitioners—for the populations most served by health departments.

With a modular curriculum, ECU could also more effectively meet the needs of health departments in their part of the state. Likewise, the UNC program saw a need for nurse practitioners with specialized preparation to serve the older population—and they secured a three-year federal grant to prepare geriatric nurse practitioners. In 1977, UNC secured funding to add another module to the nurse practitioner curriculum, a psych–mental health module—this in response to practicing NPs' requests for more knowledge about managing common and uncomplicated mental health problems seen in primary care settings. The grant, written by me in consultation with all consortium faculty, provided funding to all three programs of the consortium. The modular curriculum gave flexibility to consortium programs to adapt offerings to the needs in their areas.

The consortium did achieve the "controlled diversity" in curricular objectives and content they sought, and they did so with ease. A value-added benefit was that all three programs learned from each other, and all were better for it. But not only did the programs develop comparable curricula; they also used a common set of end-program evaluation tools. With funding from UNC's PRIMEX grant, several educational specialists were hired by the UNC program—with the intent to develop a mechanism of assessing nurse practitioner clinical reasoning by means of an objective paper-and-pencil exam. The Logic Problem Exam method was a rather technologically advanced testing method for its time in 1975.

> The logic problem [was] one method of assessing with paper and pencil the nurse practitioner's ability to 1) select data to be gathered in solving clinical problems, 2) to organize the gathered data in support of the diagnosis(es) and plan, and 3) to diagnose and establish a plan of care for clinical problems.[19]

In the exam, various clinical situations or presenting problems were described. A series of possible history-gathering questions followed. The student was instructed to select only those queries pertinent to the presenting problem. Once a question(s) was selected, the student's use of a special felt pen revealed the once-hidden response caused by the interaction between the felt pen and a special chemical treatment in the paper. In iterative fashion, the student would proceed through the history and physical exam. They were then asked to develop a plan of care. In each step of the clinical-reasoning process, multiple correct and incorrect options were presented to the student. In essence, the student's entire clinical process and logical reasoning could be determined.[20] What would be considered clunky and cumbersome today was at the time quite a unique and innovative approach to assessing clinical reasoning.

Just as the medical and nursing faculty from all three programs were involved in determining a comparable curriculum across their programs, they all were involved in determining the content of the end-program "logic-problem-method" final exam. The consortium, through its collaboratively developed common curricula and use of the same end-program final exam, went a long way to assure the leaders of the medical and nursing licensing boards and professional associations that the quality of educational programs for nurse practitioners across the state did meet common specified criteria of excellence. All this occurred before there were recognized and accepted national certification programs. But even without such national programs, North Carolina established, in essence, a statewide certification program.

The consortium functioned to 1980 but adapted its structure over time—not unusual for a mature and well-functioning group. In 1974, the "Statewide Task Force" was put together informally but carefully. Political sensitivities were diplomatically tended until mutual trust developed. Conant felt perfectly comfortable letting Booth, Pickard, and me tend to these matters. In 1975, a new dean came to UNC, Laurel Copp. Understandably, she did not know any of the people involved. Wanting to be a responsible steward, she needed to understand the agreements made on behalf of the school. Before this time, each program secured funding, but now there was a grant proposal in the works that would provide funding to all three programs but administered by UNC. Given this, the consortium had to be more formalized.

The consortium divided into two groups. An administrative group of the deans of ECU and UNC and the nursing director of MAHEC managed the consortium's more formal and financial aspects. The second group, the program group, consisted of the faculty of each program; they functioned much as they had in the past. But as each program matured, as AHEC initiatives expanded, and as the two schools, UNC and ECU, grew and developed new initiatives, the need for the consortium diminished. As Copp observed,

> One test of a true and strong consortium is if they can stand, with or without funding, and maintain some level of productivity and professional relationships when [the funding] dries up. It was there predating the funding and is there now following the funding. I feel as though the funding did not take over and change something. I feel it [the consortium] was truly facilitative.[21]

The consortium had achieved more than it set out to do. There were programs in the east, west, and central Piedmont of the state. The role and responsibilities of nurse practitioners were defined and accepted across the state and by the professional societies and legal authorities. Each program was stable on its own.

UNC and ECU began offering both the continuing education (CE) certificate and graduate degree options concurrently for several years and then phased out the certificate program option. MAHEC continued as a certificate program as there was not yet a graduate program in the west to offer a nurse practitioner program and there was still a great demand for nurse practitioners in the western part of the state.

By 1978, the consortium gradually changed its focus. There was turnover of faculty in all the programs. At UNC in particular, the School of Nursing under the new dean's leadership was reorganized. Julia Watkins returned full-time to the School of Public Health. Kit Nuckolls from MAHEC came to UNC to serve as department chair in a reorganized School of Nursing, where she would oversee the transition of the nurse practitioner CE program to a master's degree program. All programs had recruited new nurse practitioner faculty and saw departures as well. At UNC in 1978, Ouimette and Wilkman returned to full-time clinical practice; Milko did the same two years later. Williams left after the PRIMEX grant was finished to a deanship at the University of Kentucky. Nickols, a key leader of the ECU faculty, had gone on to pursue a PhD, and I did the same in the fall of 1978.

The consortium as it once was, a consortium of twenty-plus faculty, was no longer needed. Each program could stand on its own and had achieved its most important purpose of ensuring "controlled diversity" in their program offerings and graduate capabilities. The administrative arm of the consortium, which distributed funding to all three programs, continued until the expiration of the mental health grant.

The consortium had lived its fully useful life.

CHAPTER NINE

Professional–Legal Challenges and Collaborations

Despite the soundness of the nurse practitioner advanced practice role as a lacuna to health system problems plaguing states throughout the country, those involved discovered that good ideas and well-reasoned solutions were not enough. From its inception, the concept of the nurse practitioner generated controversy. Controversy emerged from every conceivable corner—the public, vested interests, and professional ideologies and territorialities, to name a few. For those who wanted to change the system, attentive and sustained political activism was required from nurse practitioner leaders and advocates everywhere in North Carolina.

The 1960s were marked by extraordinary growth in health care expenditures, in part the result of medical care inflation, but also a result of expanded medical services brought about by Medicare and Medicaid legislation. There was every reason to believe that increased demand would continue into the 1970s. Physicians and nurses were critically needed to meet the swelling demand. These concerns brought about a spate of professional, governmental, and legal studies to examine the supply, the role and scope, and the education of nurses.

Many studies focused on national issues, but some states examined their own particular needs. In North Carolina, a succession of legal study commissions investigated health care in the state. In parallel fashion,

federal agencies addressed the undersupply of health care professionals. The purpose here is not to discuss all the diverse studies conducted
during this period. Instead, we will focus on national and state activities
the professional societies of nursing and medicine sponsored, and then
look at the legal issues in North Carolina relevant to its nurse practitioner movement.

THE PROFESSIONAL SOCIETIES OF NURSING AND MEDICINE

The National Scene

Several well-known national studies at that time called attention to
health service problems facing the country. In 1963, the Surgeon General's Consultant Group on Nursing, comprised of leaders from nursing,
hospital administration, medicine, and the public, brought attention to
serious issues concerning that profession. The consultant group's findings and recommendations called for a significant infusion of funding
to increase the supply of baccalaureate-prepared nurses and improve the
quality of nursing education. Since increasing the supply of *qualified and
well-prepared* nurses was contingent on a qualified faculty, they called for
tripling the number of nurses with master's and doctoral degrees.[1] One
year later, federal appropriations funded those specific purposes.

The National Commission for the Study of Nursing and Nursing
Education, known as the Lysaught Report for its director, Jerome Lysaught, had a ubiquitous impact on nursing and nursing education.[2] Two
recommendations central to the commission's conclusions[3] had particular import for North Carolina's nurse practitioner movement. These
recommendations relate to the formation of "Joint Practice Commissions"—one overall national commission and counterpoint commissions
in each state. These commissions would address the complementary
roles of nurses and physicians, with particular attention given to various
expanded clinical roles of nurses.[4]

The commission moved quickly into an implementation phase, forming the National Joint Practice Commission (NJPC), with members nominated from both the American Medical Association (AMA) and the American Nurses Association (ANA). The NJPC held its first meeting in January 1972. Simultaneously, the commission explored states' readiness to form state joint practice commissions. Within a few months, in April 1971, nine states were designated "models" for implementation of the commission's recommendations. North Carolina was one of the nine states so chosen.[5] Just how North Carolina's Joint Practice Commission (NCJPC) set the stage for nurses and physicians to interact and plan together will be discussed later. But first, the focus here is on the national scene.

Cooperation and collaboration between the commission's nurses and physicians was evident and encouraging. Unfortunately, that was not always reflected by the words and actions of individual leaders in each profession or by their professional organizations. During the 1960s, they all could agree that there was a shortage of nurses, and that the health system desperately needed more nurses, so they worked together to find solutions to the nurse shortage. But thoughtless missteps in trying to solve other problems resulted in contentious exchanges between the AMA and ANA. In 1966, for example, an article in *Look Magazine*, "More than a Nurse, Less than a Doctor," inflamed nurses.[6] It was a story about the first four graduates of the new Physician Assistant Program at Duke University. Although the article intended to introduce the physician assistant concept positively to the public and to nurses, it missed the mark with nurses.

Even though a year later the pediatric nurse practitioner was introduced in Colorado, the Physician Assistant Program at Duke was out of the gate first with a flourish of publicity. The manner of its public introduction made nurses defensive and muddied the waters about the distinctions between the two emerging professions. Nurses didn't want to be doctors, nor did they want to be just a little less than doctors. Nurses wanted to be nurses, and they wanted to be all that they could be as nurses. They already did more than they were given credit for by other professionals and the public, and they wanted recognition for that as well.

Since the mid-sixties, nurses had gradually increased their responsibilities as new coronary care units (CCUs) opened in hospitals. Marianna Crane, in her *Nursing Stories* blog,[7] reviewed the start of CCUs, showing how important expanding nursing responsibilities were to the new CCUs' success. She quotes from the first book on intensive coronary care:

> [N]ew treatment technologies had to be used immediately in order to save lives. To achieve this goal, doctors must abandon traditional notions of a nurse's limited role in clinical decision making. Intensive coronary care is essentially an advanced system of nursing.... A CCU nurse must be able to perform...therapeutic measures by herself without specific orders.[8]

Since the AMA and ANA did not engage in any public discussions about expanded responsibilities for CCU nurses and the heightened collaboration between the two professions *at the bedside*, CCUs flourished. Without the usual confrontations among the organized bodies representing the two professions that came later, CCU doctors and nurses were free to develop and improve clinical care.

Despite the progress of nurses in CCUs, the nurse practitioner role continued to get tied to the physician assistant role—and the voices of organized nursing and medicine had to respond. In 1970, the AMA Council on Health Manpower sponsored an "Informational Conference on Physician Support Personnel." Eleven papers were presented. The emphasis in most was "the degree of independence allowed under continuing supervision." However, a summary statement of the papers reflected no degree of independence: "All agree that the physician must retain ultimate responsibility for the performance of his subordinates."[9] The AMA showed no interest in trying even to set a neutral tone.

That same year, adding fuel to the fire, the AMA adopted a position statement about medicine and nursing in the 1970s. The statement sets forth the AMA's commitment to increasing the significance of nurses as a primary component in delivering medical services while simultaneously reinforcing the physician as head of the health care team—often an inflammatory expression to nursing.[10] Barbara Bates, MD, only a few months earlier and in stark contrast to the AMA, set a more open and conciliatory tone when she suggested that "medical authoritarianism" and nursing dependence inhibited the potential of a truly collaborative team, which Bates, as a practicing physician, advocated.[11] However, the official voice of medicine did not take further note.

The AMA continued with what nurses considered rather outlandish statements. For example, the AMA proclaimed, without consulting nurses, that nurses could be trained as physician assistants, thereby plugging the hole in the dike of physician shortages.[12] These pronouncements were unambiguous: nurses would be there to serve physicians.

Nurses were enraged again, and the statements from the AMA did nothing to help nurses accept the nurse practitioner. For nurses opposed to the new nurse practitioner role, AMA statements only confirmed their worst beliefs—that nurse practitioners were mini-doctors, not nurses. Nurse practitioner advocates claimed NPs were distinct from PAs. But nurse practitioner advocates were not effective in describing the differences between nurse practitioners and physician assistants—for the public or for the nursing and medical professions. Compounding matters further, the public saw their care as similar.[13]

Holt provides a perspective on the antagonism stemming from nursing's continuing struggle as a female-dominated profession juxtaposed against a male-dominated medical profession.

The nursing profession was in the process of shaping a major transition in the image of the nurse that was as necessary as the societal transformation that was improving the position and opportunities open to women in general.... [But] organized nursing could not dissociate [from] the opinions of the AMA.[14]

Consequently, the organized societies continued to spar, in print and in public pronouncements, while individual nurses and physicians went about trying to improve collaboration and develop innovative and expanded nurse roles.

In North Carolina

During the late 1960s, the relationship between the state's medical society (NCMS) and nursing association (NCNA) was often positive, sometimes even collaborative, depending on the issue, and certainly different from that on the national level. There were contentious issues, but they did not air their disagreements in the public media. Representatives from nursing and medicine served together on various General Assembly legislative study commissions. Frankie Miller, a lobbyist and executive director of NCNA, attributes these more amicable relationships to the state's readiness to form a Joint Practice Committee based on the Lysaught Report's recommendations.[15]

Margaret Dolan, a member of the commission and former president of NCNA, kept everyone informed so that the NCNA could monitor the national commission's discussions and progress. As the national commission was nearing its final recommendations, NCNA learned that nine states would be identified as target states to implement the commission's recommendations. NCNA talked with Dolan and wrote to Lysaught, describing the existing resources in North Carolina that would enable it to develop a thriving joint practice commission.[16]

A Joint Advisory Committee on Nursing Education, advisory to the Board of Higher Education and the Board of Education, was already in existence.[17] It served as a statewide planning committee to address nursing education, one of the national commission's recommendations for study. The Joint Advisory Committee agreed to serve in the capacity recommended by the national commission (i.e., to serve as the Master Planning Committee for Nursing Education since that intent was in line with their mission). NCNA also spoke with the medical society about creating a state Joint Practice Committee, to which they agreed.

In 1971, the National Commission for Nursing and Nursing Education designated North Carolina as one of nine target states to demonstrate the effectiveness of its recommendations. Not wasting any time, a North Carolina Joint Practice Committee (NCJPC) of nurses and physicians was established in 1972 to address practice issues.[18] The Joint Advisory Committee on Nursing Education served as a master planning committee for nursing education. The NCJPC set the stage for nurses and physicians to sit together to deliberate various expanded roles for nurses and enhanced nurse–physician relationships.

At first, they concentrated on the nurse practitioner. But NCNA suggested they examine other practice sites where nurses were functioning in advanced nursing roles. So the NCJPC set up smaller task forces to study expanded and advanced nursing roles in various practice sites. Each task force brought together nurses and physicians who were not necessarily members of the NCJPC—thereby increasing the numbers of nurses and physicians who became involved in the study of nursing and consequently vested in changing nurse–physician relationships. Over the next four years, six task forces published reports—highlighting the expanding role of nurses in multiple settings.[19, 20]

The formation of the North Carolina's JPC was timely. At about the same time, a Legislative Study Committee on the Lawful Role of the

Nurse began its work. The study committee invited the NCJPC to sit in on all of the legislative study committee's meetings. Consequently, considerable issue clarification and cross-fertilization of ideas and plans occurred among the two groups.

The membership of the NCJPC was consequential. The first chair was Edgar T. Beddingfield, Jr., the quintessential medical statesman, and as importantly, a beloved family doctor—and the physician who agreed to provide backup services to the new Walstonburg clinic. For several years, Beddingfield served as chair of the influential legislative committee of the NCMS and, in 1969, became its elected president. He also served as chair of the legislative committee of the AMA. As a medical politician, his reputation was impeccable, garnering respect from all disciplines and legislators. He lent his influence and stature to North Carolina's nurse practitioner movement from early on and continued to do so while chairing the NCJPC for six years.

The leadership of the NCJPC consisted of a physician and nurse serving as chair and cochair. Allene (Fuller) Cooley, who later became a nurse practitioner, served as the first cochair with Beddingfield. Cooley was also the niece of the well-known Margaret Dolan who no doubt had inspired and influenced her niece, just as she had many other nurses. Glenn Pickard joined the NCJPC in 1971, the most informed member about nurse practitioners. I was appointed cochair in the mid-seventies serving alongside Beddingfield, and then became cochair with Pickard. Many other nurses and physicians of distinction served on the NCJPC and on its task forces. But the continuing involvement of Beddingfield, Pickard, and I allowed us to develop linkages with other medical, nursing, and legislative leaders. It kept us in the right circles when and if any threats to the nurse practitioner movement surfaced.

The National Joint ANA–AMA Practice Commission dissolved after a couple of years, unable to repair the damage from the AMA and ANA organizations' public assaults on each other. However, the North Carolina Joint Practice Committee continued to function until 1978. The NCNA capitalized on the opportunity to be one of the first states to implement the national commission's recommendations, and it turned out to be a positive force in negotiating professional and legal issues between the two professions in North Carolina.

Nurse Practitioners and the National and State Nursing Associations
Early on, the UNC pilot class struggled with defining "who they were in this new role" and whether there were any others like them. Without the internet, email, and social media, it was difficult to learn about others. According to Betty Compton:

> We [the pilot class of nurse practitioners] started to try to find other [nurse practitioners]. We asked Lucy [Conant]. Lucy helped us a lot by [referring us to] people she knew in other places who might be doing something a little bit similar, and we'd start to try to find someone who was being trained in this same way or in somewhat the same way. We started communicating by mail a lot and decided we would like—there was a large enough number—that we'd like to find ourselves a place in the organization [ANA]. I forgot who the president of the ANA at the time was, but a committee across the country was developed, out of our sort of "pocket."[21]

One by one, they found counterparts in several states, and they shared their views about a professional association to support nurse practitioners. They were unsure whether they should form a separate organization or affiliate with the American Nurses Association. The same uncertainty existed among them about affiliation with state-level nursing associations. As they wrote letters to each other, ultimately, they decided they wanted nurse practitioners to have a legitimate place in the organized structure of the national association, the ANA.

Before they made plans to affiliate at the national level with the ANA, the North Carolina nurse practitioners decided to explore an affiliation with the state nursing association, NCNA. Ultimately, the North Carolina nurse practitioners did decide to join with NCNA as a "conference group." Wilkman noted that

> Hettie [Garland] was one of a small group of people who began exploring the possibility of an interest group for nurse practitioners. They did several months' worth of work, which I was not involved in. I think probably that got started in about '71 or '72.... Basically, what we were negotiating at that time was who would be a member, providing for continuing education opportunities for people who were out in practice, providing consultation or advice or whatever to the board, to the Nurses Association, about the peculiarities of the role and who we were.[22]

They were welcomed by NCNA as a conference group. The leadership of NCNA was always supportive of nurse practitioners. According to Miller, the executive director of NCNA,

> [T]he leadership of the association [NCNA], those who are intensively involved with nursing and nursing issues, always have been [supportive].... Our board of directors, through the years, as these issues [regarding nurse practitioners] have come before the board, has always been supportive, has always felt it was one of our responsibilities to represent all of nursing. That's certainly a segment of it, and that whatever good would happen to that group is good if that happens to all of nursing; whatever is detrimental to

that group or any group in nursing is detrimental to all of nursing. They really understood and acted upon that concept.[23]

Having achieved success with North Carolina's nursing association, North Carolina's nurse practitioners, and their fellow pen-pal associates, stormed two national biennial ANA conventions in 1974 and 1976. At the 1974 ANA convention, according to Compton, the objective of the North Carolina contingent was to

> get a Family Nurse Practitioner Council. That is how it really started. After a lot of battling and negotiating and lobbying, we agreed that adult nurse practitioners should fall in the same category. There were four from New York, which were the only ones we knew at the time. And the bylaws were changed to permit the Family Nurse Practitioner Council....
>
> We could take [to the convention] all twelve [NPs] from Orange–Chatham. We worked hard. We really worked and fought hard among the delegates. When the time came, we knew our homework was done, and we knew that the vote was clean. We went out to do battle, and when it was going to be decided, we all stood around and waited. There were twelve of us probably. Between Wake, Lincoln, Orange–Chatham, Margaret [Wilkman], Martha [Henderson], Evelyn [Aabel], Agnes Binder, Phoebe [Collins], Ruth [Efird]. I mean there were twelve or more of us who were nurse practitioners.
>
> That's when I think we got the reputation of being the state that was. We made everybody think that we were doing it better than anybody else and convinced them quickly. We really did corner it.... There was a good coalition there—the two adult nurse practitioners in New York and the one in Washington, who became our key fingers on who was changing things and what was happening

in Kansas City [home of ANA's national office]. They were really vital in helping us keep it afloat, and not let the bylaws be changed for as long as possible, to make it too academic and nonpractice related.... We ended up with some real strong support from California. The nurses that were at Davis, who were in some form of a nurse practitioner program. There was such a positive force taking place that it would have been difficult to vote it any other way, I think. By the time that these twelve convinced these two and three and four, we had tremendous support for the nurse practitioner movement and a council in the ANA.[24,25]

In 1975, the ANA held an interim business meeting, and again, a North Carolina contingent showed up. "The bylaws were going to be changed again in favor of a less clinical, less formal curriculum. We were able to hold it off again. The following year, in 1976, things began to change."[26,27] In September 1975, the two councils, the family and pediatric nurse practitioner councils, sponsored joint clinical program sessions. They also held their annual business meetings separately, in which they both agreed to merge into one council, a Council of Primary Care Nurse Practitioners.[28]

Indeed, there was an entirely different atmosphere at the 1976 convention. By this time, opposition to the nurse practitioner role had mellowed as more and more nurses in education began to appreciate the clinical emphasis of their work. The tone of the official statements of ANA reflected more acceptance of NPs. The final hurdle—to bring under one umbrella family nurse practitioners, adult nurse practitioners, and pediatric nurse practitioners—had been adopted. Initially, the pediatric group held out as a separate group to preserve their own unique identity. But as the professions and the public began to understand and accept nurse practitioners, merging as one council made more sense and gave them all increased collective influence. Per their agreement during their joint session the previous year, the 1976 House of Delegates made the bylaw change official to create the broadly inclusive Primary Care Council. A decade after the first PNP program and six years after North Carolina's first FNP program, organized nursing's official position turned from overt opposition to near-unanimous endorsement.

The early graduates of North Carolina's FNP Program knew their influence was a force to be reckoned with, and so did those who worked with them at the '74 and '76 national ANA conventions. During the seventies, many of them continued to serve in an official capacity at both the national and state association levels. Margaret Wilkman, an FNP graduate of the UNC pilot class and the first nurse practitioner appointed as faculty to the UNC FNP Program, became the first chair of the FNP Conference Group of NCNA. Hettie Garland went on to serve as president of the NCNA. At the national level, Judy Roberts served on the first Executive FNP Council, and I served as vice chair of the newly merged Council of Primary Care Nurse Practitioners.

In contrast to the national organization for nurses, NCNA, the state association, welcomed them from the beginning. The membership and leadership of ANA had been critical and skeptical of the nurse practitioner movement, and nurse practitioners had had to fight there to maintain the primacy and enduring recognition of the clinical essence of their role. The same was not true, however, of North Carolina's nursing association, where NPs were favorably received.

Faculty of Nurse Practitioner Programs in Need of an Association

From the mid-fifties to the mid-sixties, faculty of nurse practitioner programs developed their curricula as they went along, some might say, "on the fly." That was true for the pilot UNC FNP Program. They, and others, started with informal, one-on-one teaching in the clinic, learning day by day what content was needed to teach nurses to become nurse practitioners. Over time, curricula became more definitive, and faculty began to share their ideas and experiences in designing nurse practitioner curricula, and teaching and evaluation strategies. But this sharing was unorganized and random—subject to meeting colleagues across the country at meetings and conferences set up to discuss matters unrelated to teaching nurse practitioners.

The three NP programs in North Carolina had the very positive experience of having a structure, the North Carolina Nurse Practitioner Consortium, through which faculty could come together with purpose to share and discuss ideas and teaching strategies. They soon wanted to share with other faculty in other states. Recognizing the value of exchanging ideas, the Division of Nursing contracted with the University of North Carolina at Chapel Hill to plan and host a conference of nurse and physician faculty from programs located throughout the country. In January 1976, UNC hosted a three-day national conference for seventy-five nurse practitioner faculty from twenty-five programs located in twenty-one states.

Day one was devoted to the presentation of papers intended to identify critical issues and to stimulate discussion from multiple perspectives. A panel reacted to each paper and comments/questions were taken from the audience. The second day was spent in group work, perhaps the most productive part of the conference. Groups were divided into areas of the nurse practitioner curriculum, as identified by participants through a preprogram assessment of priority issues. The last day consisted of summaries of group work and recommendations for the future.

The conference was highly valued by the participants—so much so that they wanted to plan for the next meeting, and to have more such meetings and opportunities for program faculty to talk with each other. In other words, just like practicing nurse practitioners, faculty recognized their need for a national organization to support their continued collective interactions and learning.[29] NP faculty continued to meet over the next few years, and in 1980, the first organizational meeting for the National Organization of Nurse Practitioner Faculties was organized.[30]

North Carolina's Legal Challenges and Accommodations

The North Carolina General Assembly was attuned to health and health care issues from the fifties through the seventies. The sting from being the state with the highest WWII draft rejection rate lasted well into the early sixties. Under Governor Broughton, the legislature moved quickly to fund new nursing and dentistry schools and expand the medical school from a two-year to a four-year full-fledged medical school. Those actions did produce more physicians and nurses for the state, but they did not solve the problem for long.

At that time, the North Carolina legislature convened in full session every two years. In 1963, they started a tradition to convene study commissions in between the full-session years. The study commissions would address urgent, and often controversial, issues so that findings and recommendations could be presented in an almost finished form to the legislature early in the next full session, so that discussion and amendments could proceed smoothly to a vote. David Warren of UNC's Institute of Government was involved in many of these study commissions.[31]

Since 1964, legislators had become aware of an increasing shortage of nurses and other health care professionals. A survey sponsored by the state's Board of Higher Education, Board of Education, and Medical Care Commission called for increased financing, statewide planning, and minimum nursing education requirements.[32] According to Warren:

[O]ut of the hundreds of legislators who had served, my point is that some of the most powerful and most political of the legislators have been interested in health, which I think explains one reason why it has been somewhat on the front burner, [in addition to] all the other reasons—nurses being interested in it, and educators being bright and politically savvy and all that, and Audrey Booth being involved. But I think the fact that some of the smartest—at least politically smartest—legislators were interested in health as an issue caused a continuing public policy debate on health in North Carolina.[33]

Since the 1964 survey through 1977, five legislative study commissions focused on the state's health care workforce. A 1967 study focused on the critical nurse shortage and recommended funds for nursing education programs and student aid.[34] Two years later, in 1969, a study commission focused on the doctor shortage in rural areas,[35] and in 1971, the focus was on physician assistant (PA) education and the legal status of PAs.[36] Then, in 1973, attention turned to nurse practitioners and their lawful role.[37] And finally, in 1977, a study commission examined both NPs and PAs, recommending amendments to the medical and nursing practice laws to legalize prescriptive authority for the two professions.[38]

All of these study commissions recommended legislation to fund medical and nursing education, and to authorize the practice of NPs and PAs. PA-enabling legislation preceded any NP legislation. Furthermore, both Duke and UNC, independently, studied the legal issues of these new health care providers—so they would be prepared to give testimony to influence the findings of the study commissions.

Invariably, in discussions about the nurse practitioner movement in North Carolina, questions surface about the PA Program at Duke University, twelve miles down the road from UNC. Such comparisons are inevitable as the Duke PA Program began around the same time, the mid-sixties, that UNC was contemplating a nurse practitioner role in its own continuing care experiments, laying the foundation for a formalized nurse practitioner program. And certainly, the "FNP at UNC" and the "PA at Duke" crisscrossed often as these new programs were discussed by nurses and physicians across the state. This was especially true when the question of legal authorization was addressed.

Eugene Stead, the founder of Duke's PA Program, was first out of the gate to study the best ways to legalize the practice of PAs—and he invited Pickard, Booth, and Warren to the legal conferences Duke sponsored on the matter. But UNC did not want FNPs amalgamated with PAs in any legislative act. For one, FNPs held their own license as registered nurses (RN), and UNC felt that RN licensure was an important distinction between FNPs and PAs. Second, UNC was fostering a different relationship between FNPs and physicians than Duke was with PAs. UNC felt that their emphasis on a collaborative NP–physician relationship was another important distinction between the two emerging professions. Third, Stead felt rebuffed by organized nursing's rejection of prior nursing experiments at Duke aimed at enhancing clinical nursing practice.[39]

Stead had been a leader in and staunch supporter of these experiments. He was a powerful figure at Duke, and thus the state as well. As a founding member of the National Academy of Sciences of the Institute of Medicine, he was also influential nationally. No one at UNC wanted to risk facing the opposition of Stead over legal sanctioning of FNP practice. Consequently, publicly, and amicably, each decided to develop their own legal positions. There was minimal to no open hostility expressed about each other's programs during their developmental years.

Legal Authority for PAs: The Duke University Position

In 1965, Duke University's Physician Assistant Program preceded the FNP Program by five years. The two programs had different origins in both time and intent. When the first class of PA students was about to finish, Eugene Stead, Harvey Estes, and others at Duke began to be concerned about the legal status of their PAs. By this time, Stead—always successful in making a case and garnering outside support for his projects—received money from the Commonwealth Fund to study the legal issues of these new health professionals. Martha Ballenger, an attorney, joined Stead and Estes, and for the next two years, Ballenger coordinated efforts at Duke to develop model legislation for physician assistants in North Carolina.[40]

Duke also sponsored a series of conferences on the legal aspect of PA practice. National health law experts were invited to present various positions and legal alternatives. Stakeholders from the state's nursing and medical regulatory boards and the professional societies attended these meetings, as did Audrey Booth, Glenn Pickard, and David Warren of UNC as noted above. According to Estes:

> [T]here was a clear feeling that licensure was not the answer.... So, we decided to steer away from licensure and to move with regulation and registration, which was what was recommended, and I think this has been influential in setting up the pattern for state laws regulating PAs all over the country. I don't think North Carolina was the first to pass it.... [S]omebody else got that first, but the model...was set in those conferences, and was very useful. The decision was made to make the practice of the physician assistant an exception to the Medical Practice Act rather than to write a licensure act, and then have rules and regulations governing what is meant by those exceptions.[41,42]

In 1971, North Carolina amended its Medical Practice Act, allowing PAs to work under the supervision of a licensed physician. Similar laws governing PAs were subsequently adopted across the country.

UNC's Position on FNP Legitimization

The Duke group thought that NPs should just follow the model that had been cut by PAs, but to those at UNC, it was not quite that simple. NPs were already recognized as licensed providers under the Nurse Practice

Act. Further, the PA "model" legislation that stipulated practice under the supervision of a physician, with the supervising physician determining the duties and roles of PAs did not sit well with nurses nor with those who had conceived of the NP role.

Before the first nurse practitioner student enrolled in the program, UNC asked David Warren of the UNC Institute of Government for an opinion on whether NPs needed specific legal authorization to practice. Warren's first opinion agreed with the position advocated and taken by UNC. According to Warren:

> [T]he original solution, as I wrote in my memo of 1968, that the nurse license law ought to be interpreted broadly enough to include nurses doing anything that they are legitimately trained to do, means if they're given extra special training as a nurse practitioner, that ought to be covered in their regular nurse's license law, not under some special, separate licensure.[43]

When the PA enabling legislation came before the General Assembly, UNC declined to join. Pickard recalls that in 1971, they had informed the Board of Medical Examiners about UNC's position regarding NPs:

> [W]e decided we didn't want to go for [the PA-enabling legislation model]. We wanted to keep them separate. There was a major policy decision as to whether to be swept in the same bag or keep them separate. We elected, for medical and nursing political reasons, to keep the two programs separate. So, we decided not to go for enabling legislation in '71.[44]

Conant and Pickard both testified before the 1971 study commission. Lucy Conant, dean of the nursing school at Chapel Hill, testified:

[T]he current Nurse Practice Act in North Carolina defines nursing broadly enough so that new activities and types of practice can be included without any difficulty. Many aspects of patient care, which only physicians performed in the past, are now accepted nursing activities.[45]

Pickard supported that view. He testified that

[T]he practice of nurse practitioners would not require additional legislation, but rather will occur through a process of evolution within existing legal frameworks.[46]

The 1971 study commission did not recommend any change to the Nurse Practice Act; their final recommendations were limited to legislative changes affecting the authorization of PA practice. Pickard had been dutiful in keeping the Board of Medical Examiners informed about the practice of NPs; without opposition from the Medical Board, the study commission accepted UNC's position on the FNP's legal status.

UNC then turned their attention to the North Carolina Medical Society (NCMS), seeking the public endorsement of nurse practitioners by that professional body. Pickard, as with the Board of Medical Examiners, also kept the Medical Society officers and staff regularly informed; he did the same with Ed Beddingfield, the former yet still influential past president of the organization. Pickard also worked with the Orange County Medical Society to introduce a resolution of NP support at the medical society's annual convention. According to Pickard, the NCMS procedure for endorsing causes can be tedious, but they felt they had done their homework. They could not be sure, though.

There was a county resolution that came in supporting the nurse practitioner, and in the workings of the state medical society, these get referred to a reference committee. You have public hearings during the state society convention for a day on all the issues. Our [resolution] came up and was hashed over by the reference committee.

I was at the state meeting. Ed [Beddingfield] was there, and several of us, and we thought everything was in good shape. The reference committee, as usual, goes into a closet to prepare their recommendations for the full House of Delegates. The next morning, we got up, cheerful and assuming that all was taken care of.... But, after hearing glowing praise for nurse practitioners, the resolution they came out with was just awful. I think it fell short of condemning, but it wasn't far short. It was just awful. Ed had gone to sleep, and I had gone to sleep, and we hadn't paid any attention to this. The damn thing was about to be debated on the floor of the House of Delegates when we first got a copy of the resolution to be presented.

Many of the things in the medical society, once they get on the floor, unless you're skillful, you can't stop them. The intent of the reference committee system is that [the reference committee is where] you get all the debates taken care of so the full house can efficiently and effectively carry out its business. I went to Ed and I said, "Ed, what the hell are we going to do about this?" He said, "I don't know. I haven't got time to worry with it. There's something else big going on." One of us came up with the notion that he, as a past president of the state society, had the prerogative for introducing substitute motions from the floor. I'm sure I didn't know that. Ed was the most skillful medical politician around, so he came up with the notion that if I would write a substitute resolution, he would introduce it.

I remember very distinctly going over in a corner of the lobby of the Carolina Hotel and taking a paper napkin, the only thing I could find to write on, and writing out the substitute resolution, which was basically what we'd introduced in the first place that had gotten gutted by the reference committee. [I] wrote it down on a paper napkin, got it to Ed, just literally a few minutes before this came up. At the proper moment when this resolution was introduced, he asked for a matter of personal favor as a past president;...he would like to introduce a substitute resolution. He completely bypassed what the reference committee had introduced, introducing instead this substitute resolution, which carried. Again, that was 99 percent attributable to his political power.... I think back then, the will of the state medical society was more important. The whole reason for doing it was so that when it came to the legislature the next year, you could say that the record is clear, the state medical society has endorsed this.[47]

As Pickard noted when he told this story, "It sure was a close call."

It is unclear who started the move to seek legislation to authorize nurse practitioners' performance of medical acts, but David Warren believes the Rural Health Program wanted legislation to cover NPs, just as there was legislation covering PAs. So, in 1972 a new legislative study commission was appointed to study the "lawful role of the nurse." Nurses and physicians had already hammered it out and agreed that the only aspect of NP practice that could possibly be subject to authorizing legislation was the "medical acts" that fell within the NPs' responsibility. But with the passage of the PA enabling legislation, questions arose about whether NPs should be recognized similarly.

The findings section of the commission report restates the primary purpose of the commission:

The primary purpose of this discussion is to examine the effect of existing legal constraints—primarily licensure—on the development of extended roles in nursing. The chief problem for the nurse under current laws is to avoid conduct which constitutes practicing medicine under the medical practice acts—or conversely, conduct that is not defined as within the realm of the practice of nursing by the nurse practice acts.[48]

The PA enabling legislation provided an exception to the Medical Practice Act. To many, it just seemed natural to take the same route for NPs.

Fortunately, Audrey Booth served on the commission as a lay member—the only nurse. She had been aware of the early development of the Nurse Practitioner Program from 1968 to the present as she was on the faculty of the UNC School of Nursing and was also the health professions development coordinator for the North Carolina Regional Medical Program (RMP). She was involved in many of the policy discussions at the university. In her RMP role, Booth found herself interpreting the new nurse role to RMP decision makers (primarily physicians and health administrators) and more broadly to nursing and the public. She was thus prepared for the many discussions and points of view that would be aired in the commission's hearings.

Because many of the RMP leadership were involved with the Physician Assistant Program, Booth said, "I saw to it that nurse practitioners got equal time whenever discussion turned to physician assistants."[49] Experienced in discussions of NPs vis-à-vis PAs, Booth was a widely recognized astute politician and negotiator, able to bring those with varied opinions together in compromise. Some called the Lawful Role Commission the "Booth Commission" because of the calm yet influential role Booth played in its deliberations.

The commission heard from a wide array of experts and stakeholders. Commissioners invited two legal scholars from other states to provide testimony (Nathan Hershey from the University of Pittsburgh Law

School and Blair Sadler, a law professor from the Yale School of Medicine). They both reviewed enabling NP legislation enacted by Idaho, New York, and Oklahoma, and they found those laws limiting the full range of NP practice. Neither the North Carolina medical nor nursing boards wanted their practice acts amended. None of the nursing representatives wanted to "slide in" under the PA legislation. Besides, there was a generally accepted premise that the Nurse Practice Act was adequate to encompass the practice of specifically prepared nurse practitioners.

A compromise was reached. The commission recommended legislative changes that would provide a legal basis for expanding the role of nurses in North Carolina.

> It accomplished this by expressly authorizing the licensing boards for medicine and nursing jointly to adopt regulations developed by a joint subcommittee of the boards to permit qualified nurses to perform a range of medical acts which may include diagnosing, prescribing drugs and other modes of treatment, carrying out medical procedures and doing other acts which are or may be considered to be exclusively medical rather than nursing.[50]

Warren, who served as staff to the commission, said: "I think it was the only legislation that could have been adopted by then because it gave the impression that each PA and each NP would be individually approved for tasks and functions that they had been trained to do."[51]

In the PA legislation, the Board of Medical Examiners has full authority to approve PAs. However, handing over such jurisdiction to the medical board was wholly unacceptable to nurses. The commission heard this, and it recommended that a "joint" subcommittee of representatives from the nursing and medical boards approve NPs. The compromise for a joint subcommittee was "acceptable" to UNC, but barely acceptable. But it had to be accepted as it was the only proposal on the table that was barely acceptable. The state nursing association and Board of Nursing accepted the agreement only because of the word "joint."

Furthermore, the North Carolina Medical Society had already approved the joint subcommittee process through its resolution approving NPs, which also stipulated a joint subcommittee of both boards. Pickard's cocktail napkin resolution, submitted by Beddingfield to the House of Delegates, proved to be critical and just in time. The Medical Society approved the resolution in May 1972, and in turn, submitted the resolution to the legislative commission in June 1972.[52] One simple word—joint—cemented the compromise.

Of course, the matter would not be settled until the requisite legislation was approved. Pickard describes the usual political follow-through when the Medical Society takes formal action.

> The rank and file of the Medical Society are officially bound by the actions of the Assembly [Medical Society House of Delegates] when it votes. Now, this doesn't keep individuals from doing their dirty work behind the scenes, but when you get around to a legislative session and hearings on a bill, the Medical Society is obliged to lobby for the official position of the House of Delegates. So, once you get them on record as favoring something, they have to, at least officially, go to bat and support it, and generally, they do. I think they're pretty clean about that. Now some of the more powerful members may go behind your back and try to influence their own local legislators. There's no question they're clean about it though when it comes to public hearings.[53]

Well, maybe. Or maybe not. Pickard continued,

I was furious when they slipped in the phrase, "It shall be admin-istered by the Board of Medical Examiners." Somebody that I thought was a key person in this scenario rolled over and played dead and assured me that it had to be. That was slipped in at the last minute, which has been the bane of our existence ever since, because that was not in the original act. The original act had the joint committee empowered to enact the rules and regulations. Old John Anderson [legal counsel to the NCMS] was the one who slipped it in there. I went to somebody like Ed and said, "Why are we letting him gut this bill?" after we fought, bled, and died to have this done. The rules and regulations were going to be promul-gated by the joint committee, and medicine and nursing would have equal voice in establishing all the rules by which this is carried out. Then at the last minute, the Medical Society—it was largely John Anderson's doing—got in that last, literally, phrase.[54]

Pickard heard about these changes—a single phrase—before they had been finalized. He talked to those he thought had a fair amount of politi-cal influence—Warren, Bernstein, Beddingfield—but to no avail. The law was enacted, as amended, to give the Board of Medical Examiners final authority.

This law has truly been the bane of existence for NPs in North Caro-lina ever since. It gave final approval-to-practice authority solely to the North Carolina Medical Examiners. Given the membership composi-tion of the Board of Medical Examiners and their varied predilections regarding nurse practitioners, they could rule at will and make the pro-cess of applying and qualifying for approval-to-practice as an NP either reasonable or cumbersome. Updating regulations to reflect current and more modern practice standards has been exasperating and ineffective.

The Nurse Practice Act has been modernized since then, and as

Warren claims, it very likely covers NP practice—just as it had in the previous Nurse Practice Act. But NP approval-to-practice is now so engrained in law and practice, under the final authority of the Board of Medical Examiners, it is hard to know how to change it. What was once considered model enabling legislation for NPs is now, in 2022, among the most restrictive laws governing the practice of NPs in the country.

However, this was not the end of NP legislative issues. One more final legislative study commission was appointed to study both NP and PA practice simultaneously as it related to prescriptive authority. Prior to the study commission, however, an interim bill was put forward by the Medical Society to authorize PA prescription and order writing. Frankie Miller, executive director of the NCNA, suggested they and the Medical Society appoint a joint committee to address this legislation, which they did. As Miller recalls:

> We had a joint committee meeting with [the Medical Society] to address that one piece of legislation. [T]he two organizations agreed that this piece of legislation was so controversial—we were fighting each other about it—that we needed to have a select group sit down and draw up a position paper that would identify areas of agreement and try to work out the areas of disagreement—come up with a position paper that both groups could endorse.
>
> During the lifetime of that legislative study committee was when the two organizations got together, assigned a group to come up with the position statement, which we did. Then we presented that to the study committee, and they were enormously relieved. Then they based the next piece of legislation on that report. The next session, they did pass the legislation, which outlines how a physician assistant can prescribe medications.
>
> We insisted that they [NPs and PAs] be dealt with separately,

that they not be lumped as physician extenders. So, the bill as it was passed says, "Here's what a physician assistant does; here are the circumstances under which he can prescribe medications..."; it finishes with that, and then it says, "Here's what the nurse practitioner..." and a lot of it is the very same thing, but at least they're dealt with differently. Anyway, that became law, but it was based on that joint effort between the two societies.[55]

The recommendations from the commission did codify the prescriptive authority of NPs.

As important as it was to have endorsements from the medical society, the nursing association's role throughout all the legislative efforts related to NPs was significant as well. NCNA used its well-honed communication networks to advocate for and help with NP legislation. They kept their ear to the ground, listening for any development that might impede or threaten NP practice. Unlike sister organizations in other states, they were advocates of and full-fledged partners in nurse practitioner legislative efforts.

Nurse practitioners in North Carolina developed an awareness of the influence of politics on professional and regulatory issues and the need to be on top of every legislative effort related to their practice. In 1972, they felt they had to accept the compromise legislation in which a joint committee of the Board of Nursing and Board of Medical Examiners would approve their practice. They did not want to abandon their newfound role. And they experienced firsthand the consequences when deals are made under the table instead.

The 1974 NP Practice Legislation's Effect in 2022
Today, in 2022, nurse practitioners in North Carolina frequently experience the restrictiveness of the 1972 legislation. Nurse practitioners are

not opposed to legislation that authorizes and legitimizes their advanced practice role. They are opposed to legislation that is under the control of medicine. This provision was not intended by the nurse practitioner advocates working on the proposed legislation. But, as noted above, the sleight-of-hand, under-the-table deal betrayed those working on a compromise provision. By this betrayal, legal authorization for the practice of nurse practitioners came under the control of the Board of Medicine— and what they giveth, they can taketh away. Some nurse practitioners, over the almost fifty years of this legislation, have been stung by the unfounded and indiscriminate actions of the Board of Medicine (or its "joint committee" acting on the medical board's behalf).

Another grating and unnecessary aspect of the current restrictive law is that NP practice authority is not based on the qualifications and education of a nurse practitioner. Rather, the NP's authority to practice is tied to a physician; without a sponsoring physician, authority to practice as a nurse practitioner is denied. If an NP changes her or his place of employment, for example, the previous approval to practice as an NP is void. The NP then must reapply for approval to practice, listing a new sponsoring physician on the application.

With the current North Carolina nurse practitioner enabling legislation, NPs are tied to physicians as never before. Under these conditions, physicians and nurses cannot be colleagues. Under North Carolina's law as it is, physicians are the ticket to legal authorization of nurse practitioner practice. There is no evidence to support such constraints to NP practice. Current law is reflective of aphorisms of long-gone eras: "Keep them barefoot and pregnant and tied to their sponsoring physician."

For over fifty years, nurse practitioners have been studied, and studied, and studied—more so than any other health care professional. The evidence is convincing. Nurse practitioners are competent, as measured by multiple criteria. Patients are very satisfied with care from nurse practitioners. Liability claims against nurse practitioners are minimal, especially when compared to other health care providers. Nurse practitioners, based on their own judgment, consult with and/or refer to other health care providers at comparable referral/consultation rates as other physicians. There is simply no reasoned justification for the current restrictions in the North Carolina law governing nurse practitioner practice.

Several attempts to change the North Carolina legislation have been met with great resistance from organized medicine. It is also important to note that, today, differences are fought in public media as well as in social media. Witness the AMA's tweet: *#StopScopeCreep*—which the AMA quickly took down after the outrage from nurses, replacing it with something not much better: "Patients win when … care [is] led by physicians—the most highly educated, trained and skilled health care professionals." But, as Patel points out, when organizations use wording such as *"choose an NP,"* physicians don't see this as teamwork either.[56] These national "proclamations" hinder state efforts.

Airing grievances in public with oppositional language only serves to emphasize differences. Instead of colleagueship there is confrontation, sometimes bitter; extreme positions are held firmly, making compromise impossible. In the seventies, David Warren gave us good lessons on getting the attention of the legislature. The legislature's posture is that both parties, in this instance medicine and nursing, must be in support of a legislative change; the legislature is not going to settle an argument between the two professions. And to get both professions on the same side, there must be leaders from each profession taking the lead, cooling the temperature, using neutral language, and finding common ground. According to Warren, legislative changes introduced by one side alone won't happen.[57]

The fact that North Carolina is among the few remaining states with restrictive nurse practitioner legislation is of no apparent concern to anyone in North Carolina except nurses. If David Warren's advice regarding the legislative process in the 1970s holds true for today and beyond, it is difficult to see how any legislative mandate could be modified by the nursing profession alone. For sure, it will take almost constant vigilance and commitment to monitor and document any malfeasant or inappropriate action by the existing regulatory body governing the practice of nurse practitioners. But most importantly, enlarging the group of stakeholders and influential coalitions, including those representing the two professions—medicine and nursing—will increase the likelihood of a successful change to and modernization of the laws governing the practice of nurse practitioners.

CHAPTER TEN

A Web of "Connections of Influence"

We're close to the story's end for the time covered here—the mid-sixties to the mid-seventies. Quite a few significant names have come up, some repeatedly. Certain critical events stand out. But a question still looms. How did an innovation so vehemently opposed by so many take hold across an entire state, and even in other parts of the nation, in five to six years? How did a few impassioned nurse practitioner champions succeed in the face of such strong obstacles?

Why were so many health and social activists drawn to UNC at the same time? What accounted for the state's acceptance of nurse practitioners, especially at a time when many health professionals opposed that role? What contributed to an environment at UNC that not only allowed but encouraged such innovations—with the AHEC and Rural Health Programs following the Family Nurse Practitioner Program? Why didn't the usual interprofessional and political challenges and considerable opposition stifle this innovation? Why was the novel nurse practitioner "movement" successful throughout North Carolina?

These are the questions Audrey Booth and I asked ourselves first, then again during our conversations with North Carolina's nurse practitioner founders and champions. Of course, perspectives varied because of the different positions and experiences of those queried, from a governor and attorneys working with legislators, to health administrators, university vice chancellors, deans, and faculty, and then to practicing physicians, nurses, and nurse practitioners. Despite these differing vantage points, three themes about North Carolina's uniqueness were dominant: the climate and ethos of the university's health science schools in the 1960s and early 1970s; the passionate dedication and activism of the movement's leaders; and the network established early by the founders and used consistently for more than a decade to guide and protect the nurse practitioner innovation.

UNIVERSITY CLIMATE

As described in earlier chapters, the sixties and early seventies were a time of great expansion of the university's Health Sciences Division. The deans of the schools were aware of the legislative mandate that funded this development: improve the health of North Carolinians by preparing more health care providers for the state.

In the School of Medicine, Dean Berryhill brought in an avant-garde group of faculty who thought differently about medical services, emphasizing what is now called primary care, the care that most people need most of the time. Even though powerful figures in the medical school felt that research and specialization should be the major emphasis, Berryhill, by his targeted recruitment, sought to ensure a balance in the school's mission between the two competing emphases of meeting the need for clinical health care services and biomedical research.

The School of Nursing started from scratch, opening its doors to students in 1951. Its first dean, Elizabeth Kemble, although new to North Carolina, knew that the first order of business was to provide the first baccalaureate-prepared nurses for the state. To serve the state well, she thought she needed to know it and its people better:

One of the first things I did was to get in my car and make the trip from Murphy to Manteo, from the western to eastern state borders, talking to people everywhere, in filling stations, professional offices, stores, and the like. It seemed to me that in no other part of the country did people have the feeling that the state university [UNC] is their university. I took quite seriously the idea that the boundaries of the university were the boundaries of the state.[1]

For eighteen years, the school grew and thrived under Kemble's leadership.

In 1968, a new dean, Lucy Conant, started a new era for the school— and her goals paired well with the new emphasis and interest in the School of Medicine. She understood the health care crisis in the country, and she knew nurses with expanded training could help alleviate the crisis in North Carolina. She was prepared to partner with like-minded colleagues in the medical school to bring services out from the university hospital and clinics to rural areas in the state where people lived and worked. And to do this fully, she was fully committed to starting a nurse practitioner program—a priority of hers.

These new initiatives in the schools of nursing and medicine were not that new to those in the School of Public Health. For the public health faculty, the health of the community was their long-standing and prevailing interest. Williams described this commitment:

I thought one of the distinctive features...of North Carolina was the fact that within the state itself we had such a tradition and history of interest in public health considerations. We had a rural environment, and yet we had a sophisticated university and resources. I think some other places have had one or the other, but we had both a state university that was sophisticated and had some sense of consciousness about what it had to do for the state.[2]

Many nursing and medical faculty at UNC held joint appointments in the School of Public Health. Those interested in the nurse practitioner movement found common-cause allies and partners among the public health faculty.

Glenn Wilson, the first director of the North Carolina Area Health Education Centers (AHEC) Program, responding to why it worked here, at the university, said:

> The circumstances in the state, the need within the university to do something about the rural poor in its own backyard, and the individuals who were involved—the deans of the school of nursing and medical school and the faculty—were willing to try and just do it because it was needed. I would argue that this is one of the best examples of health professionals dealing with a social problem and saying, "Let's don't worry about our position or your position or the law. Let's break new ground and do the best we can and watch it very carefully."[3]

Gene Mayer, the second director of the North Carolina AHEC Program, echoed a similar sentiment:

> The reasons the Nurse Practitioner Program was successful are the same set of reasons why AHEC was successful.... It was and is a state that, at least until now, has always tried to do something about its maldistribution [of health providers] when it identified it, and has tried to do things to solve problems through higher education of one type or another.... There was that broad context of a willingness to identify a problem by state officials, by health professionals, by academic people, and to say, "Well now, how can we help solve that through education and training?"[4]

Certainly, that singular, strong, and prevailing ethos of the three schools during the 1960s and early 1970s provided a rich environment for the nurse practitioner innovation to thrive. The complementary interests of the state and university and the glaring need for health care reform resulted in a fortuitous merger of forces giving impetus for major change and innovation.

PASSION, COMMITMENT, ACTIVISM

Birthing and raising an innovation are not day jobs. Nor are they a Monday–Friday job. In fact, to the founders and pioneers of an innovation, it was never only a job. It was a belief, a passion, a mission to be accomplished. Most new ideas do not see sustained acceptance without passionate advocates who ignite and protect the flame of innovation until it takes hold on its own. As Judy Watkins described it, "In those early days, there was a *'joie de vivre,'* so to speak, among the pioneer group."[5] Furthermore, successful innovations are rarely the result of only one or two passionate proponents. A few more join the movement. Then the handful entice another handful, and so on, until the movement gains a momentum of its own. Such was the case with North Carolina's nurse practitioner movement.

Glenn Pickard was North Carolina's most passionate, relentless, and dedicated nurse practitioner advocate. Repeatedly, others mentioned Pickard. Jim Bryan, the revered "doctor's doctor," said his role was *to spark* the increased responsibilities of nurses in the continuing care clinic, which led ultimately to the idea of nurse practitioners. When asked who campaigned the most for nurse practitioners, Bryan responded, "I was there at the beginning. Glenn was the horse. Glenn was the one. And no doubt about it."[6] In talking about the people who moved this innovation forward, Glenn Wilson said:

I think this program is a marvelous example of how you get things done in large institutions, particularly this one. You don't deal with the organization as a structure; you deal with individuals. You simply go from Lucy Conant to Ike Taylor, to Glenn Pickard, to Lou Welt, to Frank Loda, to Floyd Denny, and you don't have a committee of faculty studying it. It was rarely discussed in the Medical School Advisory Committee. This was something Ike, Lucy, and the guys wanted to do, so they did it.[7]

Gene Mayer echoed: "[And] there must have been some particular individual or group of individuals in the '60s who not only suggested it, but also were prepared and able to articulate it, to present it, to defend it, and to mobilize the right kinds of forces around them to then get it carried out."[8]

Glenn Pickard was the founder of North Carolina's nurse practitioner movement. He kept pushing the idea forward and urging the leadership of the medical school to listen, then to accept, and then to support the idea. Along the way, several risk-taking physicians and nurses in medicine and nursing joined. The university was where the foundation started, where the bricks and mortar were first laid.

Pickard peppered Dean Taylor, Berryhill's successor, with memos and articles about the need for a primary care emphasis in the medical school and about the development of nurse practitioner models across the country. Thus, when Lucy Conant came to the School of Nursing as dean, she found an ally in Taylor and a partner in Pickard, whose enthusiasm matched hers. Deans Conant and Taylor formalized their commitment to a nurse practitioner program by appointing a "curriculum committee" of nursing and medical faculty in 1969. The curriculum committee of 1969 morphed into the Policy Board of the Nurse Practitioner Program, an advisory board to the dean of nursing. Known as simply as the "Policy

Board," it became the hub of an ever-expanding network of nurse practitioner advocates, those who became the public face of the movement.

With the sanctioning of the program from the two deans, more faculty from the schools of medicine, nursing, and public health emerged to support and endorse the new concept. Some advocated for the idea before it was popular and participated in early curriculum planning discussions. Others taught in the Nurse Practitioner Program, and some provided hands-on support. There were enough of them to form a small but critical mass of promoters within the university—a group that grew over time. They may not have been the public face of the movement, but they are among those who had a sure hand in its success.

The nurses who signed up for the program during the first several years just *knew* that the nurse practitioner idea was a way to enhance nursing practice and improve care. Even though not always supported by their peers, their conviction about what this meant for nursing moved them to risk their careers. Once in practice in their communities, they demonstrated their value and contributions to those who were unsure that nurse practitioners were good for their communities. Furthermore, they demonstrated that care from nurse practitioners was far from second-best care; soon patients were seeking them out. The early nurse practitioners were real living forces in taking the nurse practitioner innovation public and making it not only acceptable but desirable. They were activists in action.

There were others—nurses, doctors, legislators, citizen leaders from local communities—who also took on the mantle of championing the nurse practitioner innovation. Some were more visible, stirring the pot locally, while others used their influence, sometimes a powerful influence, in state and national organizations to advance the NP concept. Their participation may have been limited in time or sphere, but their early and in some cases ongoing endorsement, support, and involvement were crucial to the growth of the nurse practitioner movement in the state. And, too, their support gave strength to the passionate and committed activists who advanced the nurse practitioner idea.

A NETWORK UNDER DISGUISE

Those involved with the nurse practitioner movement all knew there was a "network"—even though it was never called that. The network was the Policy Board, and it would shepherd the movement through the next decade. It was flexible enough to add members to its circle whenever the need arose. As the movement spread, those trying to change primary care in rural North Carolina knew who to call when. The Policy Board became the interface between the Nurse Practitioner Program, communities, professional organizations, regulatory bodies, and individual physicians and nurses.

Many of the complex issues emanating from and encompassing the program were addressed and resolved by this board. They constantly interpreted the role to applicants, to physicians in practice as well as to those who would assure backup support, to professional colleagues, to state agencies and legislators, and to the media. They were a link between the university and local activists trying to bring health care to their local communities. They crossed their own boundaries—university to community, and community to university—to seek solutions to a problem they recognized in common. And essential to the movement's success, the Policy Board was a critical forum where action plans vis- à-vis opposition and other thorny issues were developed. Its members played key roles in strategizing and implementing these plans.

In its early phases, the Policy Board was an intrauniversity group focused on bringing people from the three schools—medicine, nursing, and public health—to discuss the nurse practitioner concept, to plan a curriculum, and to define this new professional role. Its membership was originally confined to those within the university who were thinking about and talking about rural primary care and nurse practitioners.

A few of its early members became the indispensable, long-standing core—Glenn Pickard, Lucy Conant, and Audrey Booth. During the planning phase and first two years of the program, Pickard and Booth became the program's link to groups outside the university. Booth, a nursing faculty member, also held a highly visible position with the North Carolina Regional Medical Program (RMP), putting her in contact with many leaders in health care. Booth used her connections with these leaders in strategic ways, often explaining or clarifying questions about the new nurse practitioner, thus warding off any misunderstandings. Booth was also in the right position to lobby for grant support from the RMP to the nursing school for curriculum planning and program start-up funding. When she returned to the university full-time, she maintained her linkages with nursing leadership in the professional associations as well as in the Board of Nursing.

Pickard kept in contact with Geneva Warren in anticipation of a clinic in Prospect Hill, staffed by nurse practitioners and doctors from the medical center. He was also able to guide Mrs. Warren in soliciting legislative support and funding for the program through her political connections in the legislature and the governor's office. Of utmost importance, Pickard was duly diligent in keeping the leadership of both the North Carolina Medical Society and the North Carolina Medical Board apprised of the university's plans for a nurse practitioner program. Keeping as many as possible appropriately informed was consequential in keeping opposition at bay.

As soon as the pilot program got underway, James Bernstein was brought into the network—and onto the Policy Board—because of his connection with the Walstonburg community and ultimately the Rural Health Program. When Julia Watkins stepped up to be director of the

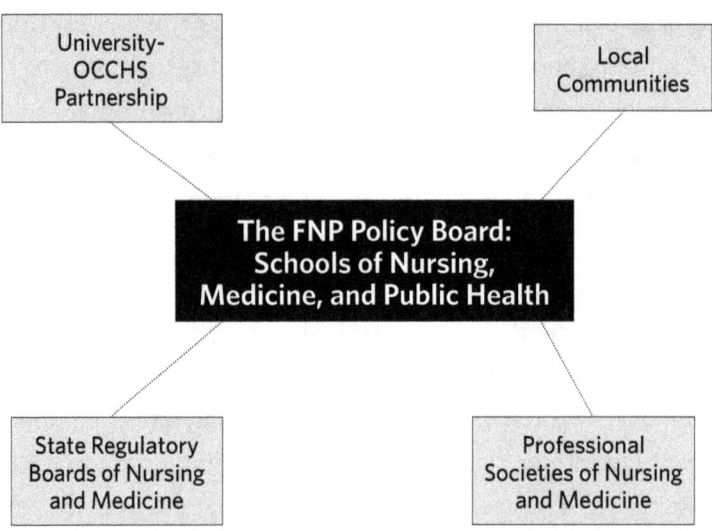

FIGURE 5. *The North Carolina NP network's early stage—1970–72.*

FNP Program, she was incorporated into the Policy Board as well. Then, when the North Carolina AHEC Program was in its early planning phases, Glenn Wilson, its first director, and then Gene Mayer, its second director, were brought into the fold. And when I returned to Chapel Hill after the satellite program trial in Tarboro, I also joined the Policy Board. Together, we were the constant and resolute foundation of the Policy Board.

The fluidity of the Policy Board's membership allowed it to maneuver both inside and outside the university. Most of the intra-university issues and deliberations occurred in the late sixties before the program started. Over time, though, it was the deliberate attentiveness to those outside the university that became paramount to the movement's success. Informal affiliations were skillfully nurtured as these relationships can be the critical ingredient when trying to influence any political process. The Policy Board excelled in tending these informal alliances and was the backbone of many important but informal coalitions.

The schematic above (figure 5) provides an overview of the groups with whom Policy Board members interacted. On first glance, the network may not seem complex, but in reality, each link to the Policy Board represented in figure 5 had multiple connections of its own, with each other, and with other groups. A final schematic presented later will illustrate the extensive and complex interactions and alliances emanating from the mature-stage Policy Board to external groups—groups whose discussions and actions have or could have direct relevance and impact on the success or failure of the nurse practitioner movement in North Carolina.

As noted earlier, initially the Policy Board existed as a "curriculum committee" appointed by Deans Taylor and Conant, and that initial action gave a clear signal of the deans' commitment to move forward with a nurse practitioner program. The interactions of the curriculum committee, soon-to-be Policy Board, were between leaders and faculty of the schools of medicine, nursing, and public health. Glenn Pickard chaired the curriculum committee. He was also the main contact between the medical school and Geneva Warren of Prospect Hill. Thus, even early on, there was contact with at least one outside local community.

As the FNP Program admitted its first class—the pilot class—other issues came before the Policy Board. For example, Glenn Pickard provided reports on his discussions with members of the Board of Medical Examiners and representatives of the Medical Society. Booth did likewise regarding the Board of Nursing and the North Carolina Nurses Association. And they all watched as the national associations representing medicine and nursing sparred with each other publicly. Already, very early in the program's development, the network extended its reach, as seen in figure 6.

Jim Bernstein, at the Health Services Research Center and School of Public Health, working with the community of Walstonburg, and ultimately becoming the first director of the state's Rural Health Program,

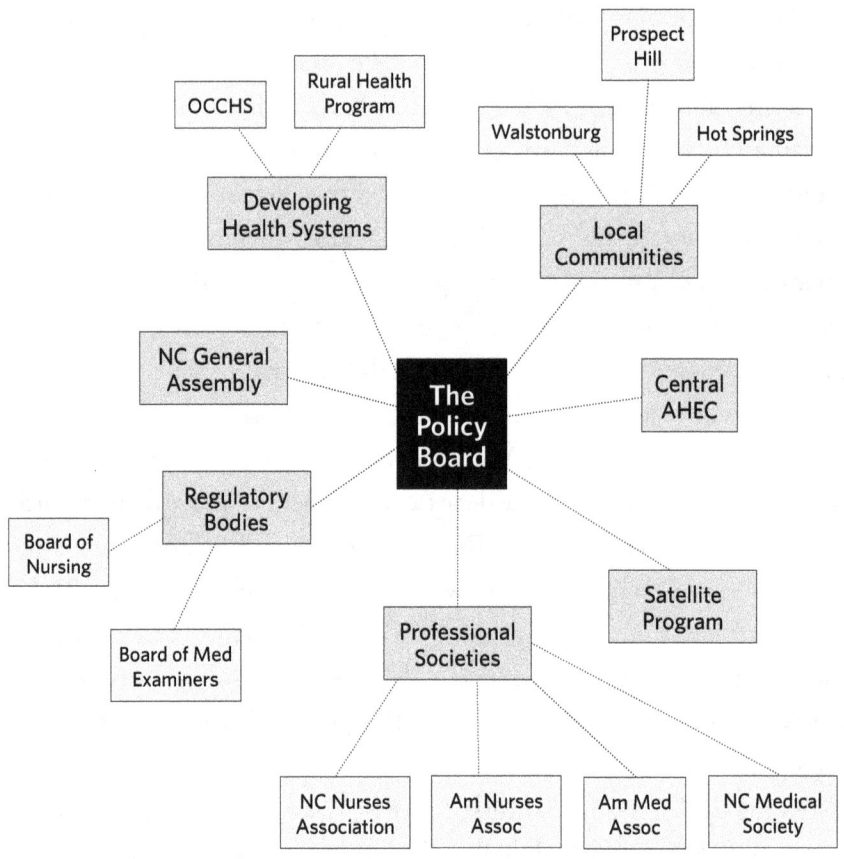

FIGURE 6. *The North Carolina NP network's second and expanding phase—1972–74.*

became a vital link to the Policy Board. He, too, formed alliances with members of the General Assembly and those in the Medical Society as he started developing rural health centers across the state. Booth was elected to the Board of Nursing and served several years as its chair—a critical position given the legislature's attention to the legality of nurse practitioner practice and, ultimately, enactment of a new amendment to the Nurse Practice Act, referred to as the "enabling nurse practitioner legislation."

The Policy Board made its final expansion when the Consortium of Statewide Nurse Practitioner Programs was established, and I joined the Policy Board. Although not every linkage, partnership, and alliance can be depicted in a schematic, figure 7 provides a glimpse of the complexity of the network that marshalled forces to make the statewide nurse practitioner movement a successful one. The North Carolina NP network, if all lines and associations could be represented, is akin to a map with Interstate and U.S. Highways, state roads, and secondary roads, all of which connect and crisscross; here we can only represent the Interstates and U.S. Highways. The best way to represent the network's central role in the North Carolina nurse practitioner movement is to give it some life—by describing some of the critical incidents in which those in the network rose to its defense in the face of challenges and obstacles to expansion.

For example, recall from the previous chapter the incident when the North Carolina Medical Society (NCMS) was about to adopt a resolution that did not support nurse practitioners, but the vote was interrupted by a substitute resolution first written on a paper napkin in a hotel lobby. When the "napkin resolution" was presented to the assembled delegates by a powerful past president of the NCMS as a matter of privilege, the substitute resolution to support NPs was adopted—just in the nick of time. However, this fortuitous turn of events didn't happen by chance. It happened because of the connections made over time and by prior networking among those advocating for nurse practitioners. Bernstein came to know Beddingfield, past president of NCMS, who then served as the backup physician to the Walstonburg clinic. Pickard had also worked hard mingling with the NCMS delegates, his physician peers, to gain support for an endorsing nurse practitioner resolution—as had Bernstein.

They all knew each other and knew they all were working toward the same end. When trouble arose, they came together to develop a

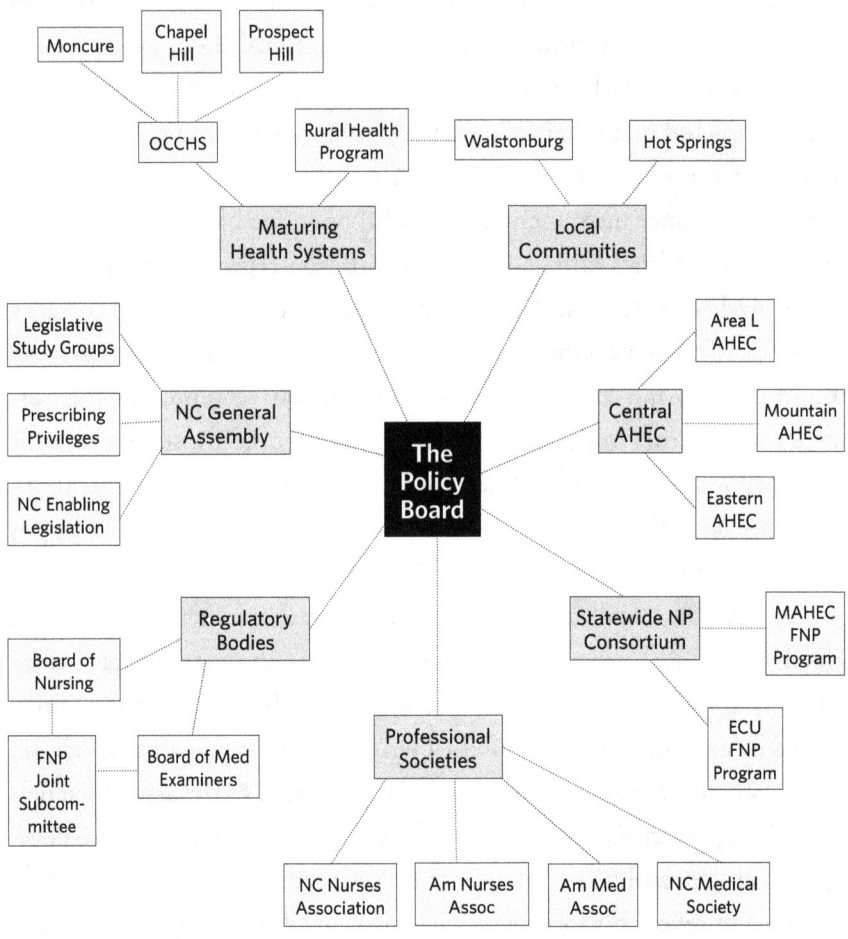

FIGURE 7. *The North Carolina NP statewide network's final phase—1974–78.*

counterstrategy that worked. Had they not known each other, had they not been in prior strategic planning sessions together, and had they not developed trust of and friendship with one another, they might not have come together that fateful day in 1972 to successfully alter the action of the North Carolina Medical Society.

Then, too, there were the times when the Hot Springs clinic became embroiled in several conflicts that had the potential to jeopardize the nurse practitioner movement in the western part of the state, and perhaps even across the state. The clinic in Hot Springs was founded independently by a public health nurse, Linda Mashburn, who saw a great need for health care services in a seriously underserved mountain community. After a difficult start, she was able to attract a physician, Robin Blake, to join the effort. By this time, Hot Springs had evolved into a three-clinic service program, with additional clinics in Marshall and Laurel, North Carolina. Blake left, though, and the clinics could not continue without some physician support. No one wanted to see the clinics in the western mountains fail, and all put their heads together to figure out a way to save Hot Springs. In the end, it was bailed out by physicians from UNC.

Glenn Pickard expressed his surprise at the willingness of the medical school to support this rescue effort. According to him:

We went to the power structure of the medical school and said, "We need some doctors up there." Floyd Denny [chair of pediatrics] and, I guess it must have been Bob Ney [chair of medicine] by then, endorsed a group of us if we were willing to go.[9]

A group of UNC physicians went back and forth, a week at a time, and covered Hot Springs for six months—an emblem of their dedication to nurse practitioners and rural primary care. Their getting to and from the west was supported by the North Carolina AHEC Program. Pickard kept the state Board of Medical Examiners informed of the effort, so that if questions came to them, they could respond calmly and informatively.

About the time of this rescue effort in Madison County, the home county of Hot Springs, the local medical society stirred up a serious issue regarding the Hot Springs clinics. The society had received reports that physicians and nurse practitioners in the clinics were engaging in illegal behavior. Glenn Wilson gave this account:

> [Apparently], a pharmacist had filed charges against [the clinics] with the Board of Pharmacy on their passing out prescriptions. We were up for illegal action. The governor had gotten excited about this; Jim Hunt [lieutenant governor] had gotten excited about this; Mr. Friday [president of the university system] thought these were good things we were doing around Chapel Hill and Walstonburg. What's this outfit out here [in the western part of the state] you guys are involved in? This was during the time Glenn [Pickard] and others were flying out there to provide backup physician coverage.[10]

The governor wanted the FNP and Rural Health Programs to succeed. So did the university president. So did everyone else. A lot was at stake.

The powerful entourage that went to the meeting in Hot Springs included not only Wilson, an associate dean of the medical school, but also Conant, the dean of the nursing school; Pickard and Watkins, FNP Program directors; Bernstein, director of the Rural Health Program; and other AHEC staff. Just as Pickard could summon his fellow physicians to fly to Hot Springs to provide medical coverage for the mountain clinics because they did not want to see these programs fail, so too could Wilson summon all the support he needed to confront the local medical society and pharmacy board. Each knew who to call for what.

When they arrived at the meeting, all the staff of the Hot Springs clinics were present, along with members of the board and many residents. A lot of accusations were flung about. Finally, the local mailman got up to speak. He told of how he had, in the past, delivered a lot of drug boxes to Hot Springs and other towns from the pharmacist who had brought forward the complaint. But lately, there were few of these deliveries. It turned out that the pharmacist who had brought charges had been filling prescriptions for patients of a physician two-years-plus dead. The mailman suspected that now more patients were patients of the Hot Springs clinics, and hence the drop in prescription refills from that pharmacist.

After this incident, they all agreed that the Hot Springs clinics needed to change their prescription protocols. They decided to hire pharmacy consultants—which they did. And the charges brought before the Board of Pharmacy were dropped.

These contacts, meetings, and the eventual resolutions weren't happenstance or coincidence. These were not the only times a local medical society, pharmacy board, private clinic, a single private physician, or a nurse stirred the pot. Every now and then, a physician in a nearby town would learn of another doctor who had brought a nurse practitioner into his practice, and the offended doctor would alert the local medical society of a problem. These issues came to the Policy Board through various avenues—someone would call Glenn Pickard or Jim Bernstein, or an AHEC office, the School of Nursing, or the medical board. In whatever way the issue presented itself, the circumstances surrounding each complaint or problem would be discussed by the Policy Board and a plan would evolve.

Usually it meant that Pickard—because it was often necessary for a physician to talk directly to another physician—went to meet with those involved. But a nurse practitioner always went with him—so that those who were raising questions or complaints could see and hear a real-live nurse practitioner. This meant that Compton, Wilkman, or I made many a trip across the state of North Carolina to meet in back rooms or small offices, often under cover of darkness. Most of the issues raised were resolved in these meetings. Issues and questions often arose because of misinformation about nurse practitioners. Simple, reasoned discussion and clarification became the salve. Meeting and talking with a nurse practitioner often helped ease tensions and doubts. Every single concern, issue, or complaint brought to the Policy Board was tended to in this way. No issue, no matter how minor, was ignored.

Sheps confirmed this commitment. "It's laborious, but you can't succeed without it. I was out at Walstonburg every six weeks over a two-year period. I went to meetings. I went out there at crucial times when they were in trouble and had to get somebody else to come in. And then I went to see what it was like."[11] Knowing that various political alliances had been made early on also provided confidence to others dealing with concerns raised from a variety of sources. Pickard gives credit to the connections made with the medical board:

> At the time we got into this, there was no question that our contacts with Bryant Galusha and Dave Citron [of the Board of Medical Examiners] were just absolutely crucial, and then through our contact with the system—and I guess that was much more in Ed's [Beddingfield] hands than in mine—Bryant got reappointed forever and so did Dave. Yes, those two really carried all the freight that needed to be carried, and we just made the multiple connections. Bryant was an AHEC physician and was in on most of the things that the group I was associated with, or we were associated with, so Bryant was part of the network, and so was Dave.[12]

So many were part of the network over time that it is impossible to name them all. As Glenn Wilson noted, "[T]he the network of bases that had to be touched regularly was just enormous."[13] And the core members of the Policy Board did due diligence keeping *everyone* in that enormous network informed and up to date; most importantly, they continually reaffirmed how important all of them were to the success of the nurse practitioner movement in North Carolina.

After 1976–77, when all the needed legislation had passed and when nurse practitioners in community clinics were more common, the Policy Board needed their external network less and less. At that time, they began to look internally, and turned their attention, once again, to the FNP Program. By the mid-seventies, nurse practitioner programs were popping up across the country. In a very short span of time, nurses no longer opposed nurse practitioners but now welcomed them. Many considered the nurse practitioner role an advanced clinical practice role. The trend in new programs became one of offering nurse practitioner programs at the master's degree level. Many certificate programs converted to master's programs, and the Chapel Hill program began to make plans to do the same—to offer the nurse practitioner courses to graduate students for graduate credit.

The Policy Board had come full circle, as it had considered this matter in 1970 in response to my petition to incorporate nurse practitioner training into my graduate program. This time, however, roles had changed. Now I was trying to persuade the physician members of the Policy Board that moving the FNP Program to the master's level was the right direction to take. I led the effort in the statewide consortium to transition the Nurse Practitioner Program from a continuing education program to a master's degree program. East Carolina University was on board, beginning its transition. But the UNC physicians were wary, fearing many competent nurses would be denied admission to a graduate program because they would not have the requisite baccalaureate degree. Further, they were particularly concerned that the hallmark of the current program, its emphasis on clinical competence, would be diluted in a master's degree program. It was with great reluctance that they conceded to a phased plan, one that would offer both the certificate and degree options simultaneously for a few years. By 1978, an FNP option was phased into the graduate curriculum, and it was more than a twist of fate that dampened the opposition to nurse practitioners among faculty, particularly graduate faculty. As Carolyn Williams observed,

> I don't think it really was until a few years ago [1978] that a conceptualization of what the [nurse practitioner role] meant in terms of nursing really began to be positively received in the School of Nursing here. You [nodding to me] were a part of that as well as Ruth Ouimette. Ruth had a big role to play in diffusing some of the negative views that had developed among certain faculty, and helping people put aside some of their fears [and] their own problems in coping with what might be a new expectation on their part.[14]

As a member of the graduate faculty, Ouimette interacted with the faculty—and they could see that their preconceptions of nurse practitioners were ill founded. In addition, Dean Copp, in 1977, initiated a total review of the undergraduate and graduate curricula. Primary care would be a major component of both curricula, and she appointed Ruth Ouimette and me to lead the task force charged with identifying primary care content for the curricula. Just as Deans Conant and Taylor's sanction helped move the Nurse Practitioner Program forward in late sixties, Dean Copp's blessing to offer the Nurse Practitioner Program at the master's degree level helped transition the program to the graduate level. In 1980, the Nurse Practitioner Program moved entirely into mainstream degree program offerings.

Nurse practitioners were accepted by the professional societies and regulatory agencies of both the nursing and medical professions. Physicians sought them out to join their practices. And, as importantly, nurse practitioners were finally accepted by faculty in schools of nursing. In less than ten short years, being a nurse practitioner was no longer considered innovative. The need for constant monitoring of opposition forces declined, as did the need for political networking and activism around the nurse practitioner role. And the need for the Policy Board and the statewide network diminished as well.

In summary, without strong community interest and support, Prospect Hill, Hot Springs, and Walstonburg would not have developed health systems that included nurse practitioners. Community support alone, however, would not have been sufficient. The support and commitment of dedicated professionals were also crucial to the development of the nurse practitioner movement, but their commitment would likewise not have been sufficient by itself. And similarly, the involvement of professional organizations and the legislature were necessary but not sufficient for the development of the nurse practitioner role in clinical practice. Only a fortuitous merger of forces led to the success of the nurse practitioner movement in North Carolina. The School of Medicine could not have done it alone. The School of Nursing could not have done it alone. But together they developed and used a network of alliances that could commandeer when needed capable supporters within the ranks of nursing and medicine.

Those comprising the nucleus of the network knew how critical it was to North Carolina's nurse practitioner movement. As Glenn Pickard noted, "Most of us involved were politicians."[15] Changing the responsibilities of nurses vis-à-vis physicians and vis-à-vis other nurses was destined to raise resistance and opposition; changing the health care delivery system was guaranteed to do so even more. In truth, sensitive political savvy was desperately needed—and was delivered through a strong, interwoven web connecting those with influence.

CHAPTER ELEVEN

2022: Fifty-Plus Years Later

Fifty-plus years ago, the nurse practitioner idea sprang forward as an innovation adopted relatively quickly, and it spread far and wide, today even internationally. Usually, innovations begin with a new idea that takes hold and is incrementally modified over time until it begins to look slightly different than originally conceived. Eventually, it is no longer considered an innovation. Such is the case today with the nurse practitioner idea.

Today, nurse practitioners can be found virtually everywhere in the health care delivery system—in primary care clinics, urgent care centers, emergency departments, hospitals, nursing homes, wherever health care services are provided. Nurse practitioners provide care to families. They focus on the care of children, men, women, and mothers, as well as older people. Some may specialize in cardiology, geriatrics, orthopedics, or one of many other specialties. Though an innovation in 1970, today nurse practitioners are well recognized, accepted, and integrated throughout the health care system in North Carolina and the nation. Nurse practitioners ushered in a new order of clinical nursing practice.

In North Carolina, the nurse practitioner idea derived from the experiments in the continuing care clinic at what was then North Carolina Memorial Hospital, a small university medical center in Chapel Hill. What existed then in the 1960s and 1970s bears no resemblance to what exists now, the "UNC Health System," with hospitals and clinics spread out in every direction across the state. Other university medical centers have done the same. They are now mega-systems that compete; such health care is big business and a big industry.

The situation is similar but on a much smaller scale for the community clinics across the state in which nurse practitioners first practiced, and for the two major statewide programs that began a year or two after the Nurse Practitioner Program. They all have grown and expanded, although not on the same massive scale as university medical centers. They have kept their community focus. Likewise, nurse practitioner educational programs look far different than they did fifty years ago. In this final chapter, we'll take a snapshot of the nurse practitioner innovation as of today, and then look back at the first days—in the context of today, some fifty-plus years later.

THREE COMMUNITY PROTOTYPES

Each of the three community prototypes who began the search for a source of primary care for their own communities in the early seventies now enjoys a stable, accessible, and comprehensive source of primary care. This is true as well for many other rural communities that, in 1970, had been in the same predicament as the three community prototypes followed here.

OCCHS to Piedmont Health Services, Inc.

In 1971, Prospect Hill was the first nurse practitioner clinic to open. By that time, the Orange–Chatham Comprehensive Health Services (OCCHS) Program had been formalized, with plans to open two additional clinics in Moncure and in Chapel Hill–Carrboro. By 1972, it was a three-clinic corporation serving residents of Orange and Chatham counties. Today, OCCHS is expanded and incorporated as "Piedmont

Health Services, Inc."—serving four counties in the Piedmont region of the state through ten community health centers. Piedmont Health offers a range of services: primary care, dental care, senior care, and pharmacy services. It is also part of the WIC (Women, Infants, and Children) program, providing supplemental nutrition to women and children under five years of age.

The providers of the Carrboro and Moncure clinics, each one of the original three OCCHS clinics formed in the 1970s, reflect a diverse but complementary team of providers, including a mix of internal medicine, pediatric, and family medicine physicians; nurse practitioners and midwives; along with social workers, nutritionists, and dentists. While the Prospect Hill clinic also has social work, nutritional, and dental providers, the direct primary care providers today, as listed on its website, are entirely physicians, and the clinic appears to be a thriving training program for UNC family medicine residents. The Prospect Hill clinic was once the proud showcase of nurse practitioners in primary care practice, but today there are no nurse practitioners working in the Prospect Hill clinic.[1]

I contacted Mr. Brian Toomey, the chief executive officer of Piedmont Health, to inquire about the medicalization of the Prospect Hill clinic. I asked specifically why there were no nurse practitioners at the Prospect Hill location. Toward the end of a half-hour telephone conversation, Mr. Toomey said that without Piedmont Health, the family practice program at UNC would have difficulty finding enough "continuity clinic experiences," a residency requirement of the program. He provided no other substantive explanation, so this, perhaps, is the likely reason there are no nurse practitioners at Prospect Hill—although Mr. Toomey would not confirm this.[2] But, with eight family practice physicians and eight family practice residents on staff, all patients at Prospect Hill are fully served by this large physician group. A few months later, I told Geneva Warren's daughter, Patricia Warren, about this situation, and she responded, "No wonder!! I always ask to see a nurse practitioner when I call for an appointment, but I'm always told none are available."[3]

This is an unfortunate loss, for it is most important that the two groups of providers, family practice physicians and nurse practitioners, learn to work together constructively and collaboratively—which, at a minimum, would enhance the residency experience. Despite the Prospect Hill location, the remaining Piedmont Health clinics continue in the mission and traditions of the original OCCHS clinics, providing a mix of physician and nurse practitioner primary care providers.

Walstonburg to Greene County Health Care, Inc.

The original Walstonburg Community Health Center, the second nurse practitioner clinic to open, still stands in its original location in Greene County. It has evolved from a single center to a corporation serving a three-county area. Greene County Health, Inc. developed into a comprehensive service organization with five community health centers, three dental health centers, and two mobile vans, one providing medical services and the other dental services. In addition, the organization provides student health services from a centrally located high school. One community health center and dental clinic are named in honor of Mr. Jim Bernstein who coached and assisted the Walstonburg community in developing its first clinic.[4] The Walstonburg clinic employs a variety of health care providers, including nurse practitioners—just as it did when it opened.

Hot Springs to Hot Springs Health Program, Inc.

An article from a 1977 issue of *Appalachian Magazine* and reprinted on the Hot Springs Health Program website provides a rich history of the Hot Springs Health Program. Linda Mashburn is recognized for her early development work in establishing the first Hot Springs clinic in the remote western mountains of North Carolina.

> "No one would have dreamed, years ago, that there would be a health-care delivery system here with a $7 million annual budget and 130 to 140 employees," says Hot Springs Health Program medical director Dr. F. B. "Chipper" Jones. "We couldn't even conjure it up."[5]

The Hot Springs Health Program serves Madison County and surrounding areas. The program has four clinics and four pharmacies; in addition to comprehensive primary health care, it offers physical therapy, behavioral health counseling, and home care and hospice services. Nurse practitioners are key members of the Hot Springs Health Program. Even though the roads to and from Asheville are better now than they were in 1970, the Hot Springs Health Program provides needed and desired services to residents scattered throughout the mountainous counties of western North Carolina.

SIBLING PROGRAMS

Within a couple of years after the start of the Nurse Practitioner Program, two "sister" programs developed—each with the intent of improving and expanding access to health care services for the state's rural population. The three programs—FNP, AHEC, and Rural Health—worked collaboratively, as they shared similar objectives. They were innovative in the 1970s and became well-known across the country as many visitors were welcomed to North Carolina to observe the work of each of these programs. They all developed successfully and continue to serve North Carolina.

The North Carolina. AHEC Program started in 1972 with three regions—one of which was the Area L AHEC, where the first satellite FNP program was initiated. By 1975, nine regional AHECs were open.

Today, the AHEC Program has grown fully into its mission of supporting education and services that focus on primary care in rural communities. Clinical experiences for health professional students in rural areas are facilitated, and continuing education programs for practicing health professionals are offered locally and online. They help recruit, train, and retain the health care workforce needed in North Carolina, as was the intention of the AHEC Program at its inception.[6]

In 1973, North Carolina was the first state in the nation to create an Office of Rural Health, with the goal of focusing on the needs of the state's rural and underserved communities. The purpose of the rural health program was to provide technical assistance and start-up funding to rural communities so that each community could develop and operate its own local health service agency or center. As of 2019, seventeen designated rural health centers provided services to thirty-eight counties in the state.[7]

NURSE PRACTITIONER EDUCATION

The founders of the UNC Family Nurse Practitioner Program in 1970 had several broad yet interrelated goals. One was to offer an educational program to prepare nurses for a more advanced practice role as nurse practitioners. In 1970, the founders did not use the "advanced practice role" terminology, nor was the term used by the nursing profession at the time. But the early FNP advocates were convinced that nurses had a depth of knowledge, by both education and experience, to enable them to take on a greater scope of responsibilities in providing needed primary care services. The FNP Program was developed to provide nurses with additional knowledge and experience, preparing them for an advanced clinical role in primary care.

A second goal was to help alleviate the state's lack of rural health care services by assuring that prepared nurse practitioners would be available in needed areas across the state. A third goal was to offer nurse practitioner educational programs at several sites across the state, making nurse practitioner programs more accessible to nurses living throughout the state. They succeeded in all three of these goals within five years of the beginning of the UNC program. And, to a great extent, the programs in North Carolina and across the country continue to achieve these goals.

Access to Nurse Practitioner Educational Programs

Since the 1970s, the number of nurse practitioner programs across the country has skyrocketed. And they have changed dramatically as well. In the early '70s, most early programs were offered as continuing education programs to shelter them from faculty opposed to these novel programs. Some of the early opponents of nurse practitioners may have thought the new programs to be inferior—but their assumptions were proven wrong. These programs required one full year of full-time study, following basic education as a nurse and several years of practice. They were planned by physicians and nurses collaboratively. Graduates passed national certification exams when those were eventually developed.

In 1977, it was time to plan the transition from a certificate-granting nurse practitioner program to a mainstream, degree-granting program within the School of Nursing. Two years later, this transition occurred; UNC's Nurse Practitioner Program was offered as a master's degree clinical option. Some expressed concern about this change, fearful that many competent nurses would be prohibited from becoming nurse practitioners because they did not have the requisite baccalaureate degrees. Most importantly, they worried whether the same magnitude of emphasis on clinical competence in the certificate program would carry through to the master's program. As it turned out, these fears, although understandable, did not materialize.

Educational accessibility has changed and expanded in remarkable ways since the 1970s as well. Multiple pathways are now available for nurses to change their career focus after years of experience or to increase their educational backgrounds after their initial nursing degree. Today, nurse practitioner programs are offered at the master's and doctoral levels, leading to MSN (Master of Science in Nursing) and DNP (Doctor of Nursing Practice) degrees. The many routes for those who want to become nurse practitioners include accelerated programs, post-degree programs, online options, and direct pathways from BSN to DNP degrees—and any number of combinations of the above, including programs specifically designed for nurses with diplomas and associate degrees.

While these multiple pathways were intended to provide seamless access to educational advancement, novices to the field often find the array of offerings dizzying. Yet, today, educational accessibility, in and of itself, is not the issue it once was in 1970. In its wake, however, the plethora of pathways to become a nurse practitioner has muddied the expectations for the clinical competence and role of graduates from different degree programs.

The Degree Muddle Conundrum

The lack of degree differentiation, both in curricular requirements as well as in graduate role expectations, is not a new predicament for the nursing profession. In 1965, the American Nurses Association (ANA) adopted the position that the entry degree for all "professional nurses" be the Bachelor of Science in Nursing (BSN), and that an Associate Degree in Nursing (ADN) be the entry degree for "technical nurses." Even though curricular requirements differed between the ADN and BSN degree programs, the expectations and roles of graduates from the different programs remained the same. Graduates from both programs took the same licensing exam and, upon passing it, worked as registered nurses.

Around the same time, the early sixties, the NLN would not accredit a master's degree program at Duke University designed to prepare advanced clinical practitioners because it was too clinically oriented.[8] Eventually, the profession, and the NLN, did an about-face, requiring that all master's degree programs be clinically oriented. In the instance of the Master of Science in Nursing (MSN), clear degree differentiation was achieved. For many years, the purpose of the Master of Science in Nursing degree was to prepare clinical practitioners for advanced nursing practice. Graduates were known as advanced practice nurses (APN). They were clinical specialists, nurse practitioners, nurse anesthetists, and nurse-midwives. There was, in this instance and at that time, congruence between degree requirements and role and practice expectations.

Then, in 2004, the American Association of Colleges of Nursing (AACN) recommended that all schools of nursing phase out master's level preparation for APNs, replacing master's programs with the Doctor of Nursing Practice (DNP) degree—even though the DNP purpose was to prepare APNs for *leadership* in clinical practice. Once again, the waters were muddied. Sixteen years later, APNs are prepared at both the master's (MSN) and doctoral (DNP) degree levels, with little differentiation between the clinical requirements of the two degrees and, most importantly, little differentiation in the work of the graduates of the two programs. And again, graduates of both master's and doctoral degree programs sit for the same certification exam.

So today, the nursing profession faces a dilemma like the one they faced when the early nurse practitioner programs began. Degree muddle was precisely what the early North Carolina nurse practitioner programs tried to avoid. They were successful in this, through the Consortium of Nurse Practitioner Programs, for their first ten years, but by 1980, there were many national nurse practitioner programs, and most were offered at the master's degree level by that time. But with the introduction of the DNP degree, the differences between master's- and doctoral-prepared nurse practitioners became blurred, and they have been ever since.

Despite the ubiquitous acceptance of the nurse practitioner innovation by the public and the nursing profession, and broad acceptance by practicing physicians, "degree muddle," or lack of degree differentiation, continues to plague the profession. This vexing problem was initiated and is sustained by the nursing profession itself. Today's issues are not unlike the issue it has grappled with regarding degree requirements for the basic practice of nursing for the last century and well into this century.

Recently, McCauley, et al.[9] threw down the gauntlet to their colleagues, saying it was time to reevaluate and readjust the call for a universal DNP for all advanced practice nurses. Among other recommendations, and in context here, the authors call for clarity about the education and roles of DNP graduates. The need to differentiate competency outcomes—clinical, scientific, leadership, or otherwise—of MSN and DNP graduates is critical for students, the public, and health care systems. The authors state that the transition from preparing advanced practice nurses at the master's level to a universal DNP degree was a "heavy lift" for the profession. However, there is an even heavier obligation for the profession to move from degree muddle to degree differentiation.

THE FIRST SEVEN AND THE THOUSANDS THAT FOLLOWED

On the first day of the North Carolina Family Nurse Practitioner Program, September 8, 1970, seven nurses anxiously waited to hear more about what they had signed up for. They were told they would help alleviate a rural health crisis in the state. They were told that they would change nursing practice and that doctors and nurses would now work together, relating to one another differently. They were told they were pioneers and risk takers. They were that, and in time they did all that they'd been told they would do.

But likely, they never thought on that first day that the experiment they were embarking on would turn out to be not just a state, but a national, movement. They did not anticipate that one day nurse practitioners would be working throughout the health care system. Nor did they realize what they would be contributing to nursing and to the nursing profession, and to women in nursing.

Over the course of the first six months of the training program, the pilot class spent a lot of time talking with each other about who they were as nurse practitioners and what practice would be like. Today, those aspiring to be nurses already know what a nurse practitioner is—some do even before they start nursing school. In fact, many start their first year of nursing school knowing they will go on for advanced degrees as nurse practitioners.

2020s: The Status of Nurse Practitioners

Booth and I held our interviews and conversations with North Carolina's nurse practitioner movers and shakers in the early 1980s, when a surplus of physicians was projected. Thus, when we asked about the future for nurse practitioners, some responded with doom and gloom—forecasting the end for nurse practitioners, just because there might be a physician surplus. Yet, as we see today, nothing is further from the truth. Others pointed to additional areas of unmet health care need and new opportunities for nurse practitioners beyond what had been conceived originally. These latter sentiments were much closer to the truth.

During the 1970s and 1980s, the dominant questions regarding nurse practitioners revolved around four themes. Will NPs improve patients' access to needed services? Will patients accept treatment by NPs alone? Will the clinical work of NPs generate enough revenue (i.e., be productive enough) to ensure viability of their practice and the clinics or services for whom they work? And will the quality of care provided by NPs be first rate, as opposed to second best, and will it be equivalent to care provided by physicians?

In 1986, Ostwald and Abanobi, in writing about the future of nurse practitioners, noted: "After 20 years of primary care services, the questions asked are no longer about their cost-effectiveness, the quality of services, or, for that matter, their viability."[10] A decade later in a comprehensive review of research about nurse practitioners from 1965 to 1991, I also came to a similar conclusion. "Findings confirm that nurse practitioners, in all types of settings, and with various patient populations, provide care and services that lead to positive patient outcomes; in many instances, when compared to physicians, nurse practitioner outcomes are better."[11] In the 1990s, some resistance from physicians continued, based on fears of encroachment. But today, more and more physicians find that nurse practitioners enhance the quality of services. And the public agrees.

Once just an idea, nurse practitioners are now an ongoing phenomenon. In North Carolina, in 1970, seven nurse practitioners entered practice in primary care settings in rural, underserved areas of the state. By 1975, UNC had trained 101 nurse practitioners for the state. Toward the end of the decade, by 1978, three hundred nurse practitioners were distributed throughout the state, prepared by the three programs of the consortium—UNC, ECU, and MAHEC. No small feat—having started with only seven in 1970.

Nurse practitioner growth has been exponential ever since—across the state and the nation. In 2010 there were 106,000-plus nurse practitioners in the United States. Ten years later, the number of nurse practitioners in the United States had nearly tripled; 90 percent of the 290,000 nurse practitioners in the country in 2020 were certified in primary care.[12] Future projections follow a similar growth pattern. In a 2018 article published in *The New England Journal of Medicine*, Peter Auerbach reported that the majority of health care providers joining the U.S. workforce by 2030 will be nurse practitioners or physician assistants. He goes on to report that the number of nurse practitioners will grow by 6.8 percent, compared to a growth rate of 4.3 percent for physician assistants and 1 percent for physicians. The author concluded that the influx of nurse practitioners will reshape primary care.[13]

"Boundary Shifting" Progress at Last

Despite these favorable predictions about the need for and thus, opportunities for nurse practitioners, there continues a nagging question about who controls the practice of nurse practitioners. This issue is seen differently by each profession. The body politic of medicine sees it as a problem, referring to it as "scope creep." The nursing profession, however, views the issue as a matter of professional dominance by one profession (medicine) over another (nursing).

Independence, autonomy, subservience, or collaboration—which shall it be? Within the broad field of health care, the boundaries of physicians have been limitless while the bounds of other health care professionals have been limited. The practice boundaries of other health care professionals are defined, by law and custom, in relation to the rigidly defined and assiduously guarded boundaries claimed by the medical profession. In other words, the determination of the scope of practice of other health care professionals is measured solely against the legally defined scope of medical practice. However, when physicians no longer choose to bear responsibility for some aspect of their practice, they merely pass that responsibility on to some other health professional. Then, at their convenience, their strictly drawn lines protecting their practice fade away. As noted previously, this has been true for at least the last century.

In 1970, in North Carolina, the Family Nurse Practitioner Program developers adamantly claimed that NP practice was a natural and continuing expansion of nursing practice based on additional education, and because of this, NP practice fell within the scope of the state's Nurse Practice Act. However, counterforces emanating from medicine claimed otherwise. Two years earlier in 1968, in North Carolina, PA practice was legalized as an exception to the Medical Practice Act—which of course allowed physicians to maintain tight control over PA practice entitlements. Consequently, incorporating legal authorization to practice as a nurse practitioner under the Nurse Practice Act was a battle lost before it even began. And so, NP practice in North Carolina was also legally authorized as an exception to the Medical Practice Act, just as had been done for PAs.

When authorizing legislation for nurse practitioners was enacted in 1972, it was considered one of the most advanced pieces of legislation governing nurse practitioner practice, likely only because North Carolina was one of the early states to adopt any NP-related legislation. And usually, any legislation enacted first is likely to be conservative. Nonetheless, as more states adopted NP-authorizing legislation, they learned of North Carolina's problems with its legislation, and they made modifications, further refining the tenets of their own states' legislation in less restrictive language. In 2022, North Carolina's legislation was among the most restrictive legislation affecting nurse practitioners' scope of practice in the country.

Fortunately, today, there is a new movement afoot. The Robert Wood Johnson Foundation, along with the AARP Foundation and AARP, in 2010 founded the Future of Nursing: Campaign for Action. One goal of the Campaign for Action is to remove legal barriers that prevent nurse practitioners from providing care to the full extent of their education and training.[14] In 2021, the Campaign for Action reported that all but eight states made progress in removing legal barriers to nurse practitioner practice; unfortunately, North Carolina is among the eight states that have made no progress to remove legal restrictions.

Boundaries exist to limit and to control. Boundaries inhibit rather than encourage collaboration, something vital to all practicing professionals.

And importantly, the public's access to quality health care services is not well served by such tightly controlled boundaries.

For over a decade during each legislative session, the nursing profession and its allies have attempted to change North Carolina's legislation governing NP practice, but powerful and monied forces from medicine have fought such changes. Nearly a dozen nurses have been elected to North Carolina's legislature, serving as a voice of authority and legitimacy about nursing practice issues, but their voices are lost amid the domineering shouts from medicine and the generous support of legislators by the monied lobbyists of medicine. As discussed in previous chapters, there is absolutely no evidence supporting legislation that serves to restrict the scope of nurse practitioner practice, nor is their any evidence to suggest that the practice of nurse practitioners should be governed by any group other than the State's existing nursing regulatory body.

I held back the publication of this book for close to two months while the N.C. General Assembly considered, once again, legislation to grant NPs full practice authority (the SAVE Act). The bill made it through two votes in the Senate with only 2 no votes, leading the nurse legislators, state nursing association, and large coalition of NP allies thinking this might be the year that the N.C. legislature would remove legal barriers to nurse practitioner practice. They also knew there would be a battle in the House.

The bill was held in committee and thus was stalled in the House. Toward the final hours of the session, N.C. Representative Gale Adcock, an FNP, filled a discharge petition—a bold and creative maneuver to bring the bill out of committee for a floor vote, where a supermajority would support the bill. Medical lobbyists panicked—until the House speaker pulled the bill out of the Health Committee and sent it to the Rules Committee, where it languished until the session was over. Organized medicine's "deep pockets" bolstered the House leadership to block the move for a floor vote.

As reported by several news outlets, and confirmed by Representative Adcock, despite bold political maneuvering, support from a supermajority of legislators, and a strong coalition of allies, money and campaign contributions talked louder.[15] But nurses, nurse practitioners, organized nursing, and their growing coalition of supporters are emboldened and looking forward. The real fight for full practice authority for nurse practitioners and advanced practice nurses in N.C. has only begun.

The North Carolina Nurse Practitioner Collection: Conversations with the Movement's Influentials[1]

INTRODUCTION

The University of North Carolina at Chapel Hill (UNC) School of Nursing started its Family Nurse Practitioner Program in September 1970. That date marks the beginning of the nurse practitioner movement in North Carolina. However, other related events preceded this important marker that also inspired and influenced the early development of the state's nurse practitioner movement. In the late 1960s, several experiments to expand the role and responsibility of nurses occurred at both UNC and Duke University—and any history of the nurse practitioner movement in North Carolina would be shortsighted without reference to these experiments.

At the same time, local leaders stepped forward to help their home communities find a new source of health care as family doctors retired. Concurrent with the second and third year of the Family Nurse Practitioner (FNP) Program at UNC, two other important health care and health education initiatives began—the North Carolina Area Health Education Centers (AHEC) Program and the North Carolina Rural Health Program. All three of these programs—the FNP Program, the AHEC Program, and the Rural Health Program—changed the landscape of both health professional education and health care delivery in North Carolina.

During the early years of the program, a small, close-knit group served as a nucleus, setting a strategic direction for the emerging nurse practitioner (NP) movement as well as troubleshooting arguments and impediments put forth by opponents and naysayers. This core group guided the NP movement's early evolution. The group knitted a robust and durable web of interweaving and ever-expanding "connections of influence" with many relevant health care leaders and organizations to advance and gain acceptance for nurse practitioners among nursing and medical professionals, communities, politicians, and would-be and actual patients. Many of these influential women and men were simultaneously involved in the Nurse Practitioner Program at UNC as well as with the developing AHEC and Rural Health Programs. In many says, these three grew up as sister programs.

How North Carolina's nurse practitioner movement started and developed is unique, and we (Cynthia M. Freund and Audrey J. Booth) felt that much could be learned about major social change from these experiences, especially in replicating similarly useful public health programs. Many of our conversation sources were notable figures in the history of health care and education in North Carolina, often as initiators of progressive forms of health care and education in the state. Examples include Ed Beddingfield, Jr., Jim Bernstein, Audrey Booth, Jim Bryan, Lucy Conant, Cynthia (Cindy) Freund, Governor James Holshouser, Eugene Mayer, Glenn Pickard, and Glenn Wilson, to name a few. Their interviews will have lasting historical value.

The chief purpose of the *Conversations Collection* was to serve as primary source material for a book describing the founding and early evolution of the nurse practitioner movement in North Carolina—and, indeed, they have served that purpose. *A New Order of Things: Origins of a Nurse Practitioner Movement* was completed in 2021. The intent of documenting the history of the NP movement was not to write a historical volume. Rather, we wanted to tell the story—the story of how the nurse practitioner movement came to be. We wanted to ask and record the personal answers to several questions. Why did this movement occur in North Carolina? Why did a handful of people who were so passionately committed to common goals come together at a certain time and at a certain place? What made North Carolina right and ripe for such an innovation? What made it successful?

THE CONVERSATIONS

We conducted most interviews and conversations included in the *Freund–Booth North Carolina Nurse Practitioner Conversations Collection*[2] between 1982 and 1984,[3] four to six years after our involvement in the University of North Carolina at Chapel Hill Family Nurse Practitioner Program. Booth became involved with the University of North Carolina Family Nurse Practitioner (FNP) Program around 1968 when she became a faculty member of the UNC School of Nursing. At that time, she served as coordinator of health professions development with the North Carolina Regional Medical Program (NCRMP) and oversaw several NCRMP-funded projects enabling development of the evolving FNP Program.

In her NCRMP role Booth interacted with nurses and physicians across the state, giving her the opportunity to describe and promote ideas and concepts valuable to the Nurse Practitioner Program in the making. These relationships served her and the FNP Program very well in later years when delicate legal and interprofessional issues were negotiated. Several years later, in 1973, Booth served as the AHEC (Area Health Education Centers) director of statewide nursing activities.

I enrolled in the UNC School of Nursing master's program in 1970. Unable to combine FNP training with my master's degree requirements, I began to work closely with C. Glenn Pickard—the founding director of the FNP Program. As I worked with Pickard and his physician colleagues to learn FNP skills informally, I vicariously learned about the political maneuverings involved in getting the FNP Program off and running, and also about all the progress and setbacks encountered during those first two years. In January 1971, I conducted my graduate thesis at the Prospect Hill clinic—one of the first studies of the graduates of the new FNP Program in one of the first FNP clinics established in North Carolina.

In 1973, I went to the Area L AHEC in Tarboro, North Carolina, to establish and test the feasibility of satellite FNP training programs in rural areas while simultaneously completing my formal training as an FNP and earning national certification as an adult nurse practitioner. A year later I returned to Chapel Hill and became a full-time faculty member as associate director of the School of Nursing FNP Program as well as the AHEC coordinator and liaison of statewide FNP programs. I remained in these positions until 1978 when I left UNC to return to graduate school.

Thus, from 1968 through 1978, Audrey and/or I had many interactions with all the people interviewed later in the early 1980s. We and those we worked with and ultimately interviewed were passionate about creating a new role for nurses as a way of improving health care delivery and advancing nursing practice. When we embarked on interviewing our past colleagues, we did not intend to conduct dispassionate, neutral interviews—nor could we if we had tried. When one listens to the tapes or reads the transcripts, it can appear that friends are sitting together talking about how it all happened and relishing the past because of a shared passion for what we and they accomplished for the NP movement. During the interviews, the laughter shows that we knew the "interviewees" quite well.

On other occasions we provided a stimulus to jog the interviewee's memory; or we provided an answer when someone couldn't remember or pin down a date or a name. In other words, we were having conversations as conversations go.[4] For many, we had already proven our trustworthiness with those we interviewed—which contributed to more frank and open discussion. Because we knew as much as we did about the beginning of the NP movement in North Carolina and in the country, and because we were "coconspirators"—if you will—in driving the movement forward, we could probe for responses as needed. We knew our agenda for each influential source.

The interviews in the *Conversations Collection* are "unstructured interviews," although as noted above they were frequently conversations, and that is why the *Conversations Collection* is subtitled "conversations with." In an unstructured interview, a conversational approach is used; the conversation is guided by the interviewer, but it can change direction as the interview progresses—depending on where the conversation goes or how the interviewer decides to steer it. We did not consider this project an oral history project. At the time, neither of us was aware of the oral history field of study, thus we were not prepared by training to undertake an oral history project.

We contacted each person first by letter, explaining that our objective was to query and elicit recollections of their role in and perspective of the NP movement in North Carolina, with our stated intent to write a book about the movement. We scheduled a time and place to meet with each person, and we and they acknowledged the purpose of the meeting. We also told them we would use material from all the interviews in our book, and that we might send all the material we had gathered to a university archive or nursing history center. Before the discussion started, we answered all their questions.[5]

We had a clear plan in mind regarding the focus and goal of the discussion, using a broad written "guide" to assure that all the major points were covered. Questions posed were open-ended, with probing when needed in response to what the interviewee had said. We and each influential were "conversational partners." In the *Conversations Collection*, rapport with interviewers was established quickly because the interviewers and interviewees had known and worked with each other for several years. We had been allies and compatriots. In fact, prior to recording the interviews, the meeting often started with initial informal "catch-up" conversations. All but one interview was recorded.[6] After the interview, we sent each interviewee a letter of thanks. The interview guide, and "request for interview" and "thank you" form letters, are included as attachments to this appendix.

In the mid-1980s, Booth had the original audio tapes transcribed using the cumbersome technology of the day. She was able to verify at that time some of the names and places mentioned in the tapes. Twenty-five years later I had the audio-cassette recordings converted to MP3 digital files. I hired professional transcriptionists to transcribe the audio files to digital Word and PDF files. The transcripts were edited according to standard guidelines, using a three-pass editing process. I completed all the third-pass edits. The purpose of editing transcripts was to reflect the context and content of the interview while capturing the narrator's character and feelings. In addition, editing corrected the inevitable changes in verb tenses and the dropped words that occur naturally in conversation. A list of the interviewees in the *Conversations Collection* follows, providing a brief glimpse of the richness of some of the original source material used to describe the development of the nurse practitioner movement in North Carolina.

The original 1985 transcripts and the later MP3 files and digital transcripts are all part of the *Conversations Collection*.[7] Also included in the *Conversations Collection* are a copy of the discussion guide developed in 1982; a scanned copy of the typical letter sent to interviewees requesting an interview; and a scanned copy of the typical letter sent to interviewees thanking them for discussing the nurse practitioner movement with us and requesting their curriculum vitae and any further material of interest and usefulness to our project. This material as well as work-sheets tracking requests for interviews, dates scheduled, and follow-up issues are included with the *Conversations Collection* material, as part of the Freund Papers at the Barbara Bates Center for the Study of Nursing History, University of Pennsylvania.

ATTACHMENT 1: LIST OF INTERVIEWEES

The Influential Interviewees	*Position at Reference Time Period: 1965–78*
Bernstein, James (Jim)	Founding director of the North Carolina Office of Rural Health
Binder-Weisinger, Agnes	Graduate of the 1972–73 FNP Program and one of the early FNPs to work in a private physician group practice
Booth, Audrey	Director of health professions education, North Carolina Regional Medical Program; director of nursing activities, North Carolina AHEC Program; member and chair of the Board of Nursing; and member of the Board of Medicine/Board of Nursing Joint Subcommittee on FNP Practice
Bryan, James	Lead physician in the UNC continuing care clinic where an "expanded" nursing role was demonstrated as a precursor to the formal Nurse Practitioner Program
Compton, Betty	One of the first FNP graduates; practiced at Prospect Hill clinic, one of the first NP clinics in North Carolina
Conant, Lucy**	Dean, UNC School of Nursing (1968–75); started the FNP Program during her early tenure as dean
Copp, Laurel	Dean, UNC School of Nursing (1975–89), succeeding Dr. Lucy Conant; oversaw the transition of the FNP Program to a master's level program
Estes, Harvey	Chairman, Department of Community and Family Medicine, Duke University

Freund, Cynthia (Cindy)   Director of the first FNP satellite program in the Area L AHEC; associate director of the UNC FNP Program; and AHEC coordinator of statewide FNP programs

Garland, Hettie   First director of the FNP Program at Mountain AHEC

Greenberg, Bernard (Bernie)   Dean, School of Public Health

Holshouser, James (Jim)   Governor of North Carolina who started the North Carolina Rural Health Program

Ingles, Thelma**   Faculty, Duke University School of Nursing; collaborator with Wilson and Stead in Duke nursing practice experiments

Johnson, Betty Sue   Director of the UNC School of Nursing Graduate Program

Lawler, Terry   First director of nursing activities at Eastern AHEC; also, faculty at ECU School of Nursing and director of the ECU School of Nursing FNP Program

Mashburn, Linda   A nurse and community activist who brought the first FNPs to practice in the Hot Springs clinic in the mountains of North Carolina

Mayer, Eugene (Gene)   Associate director and then second director of the North Carolina AHEC Program

Miller, Frankie   Executive director, North Carolina Nurses Association

Nuckolls, Katherine (Kit)   First director of nursing activities at Mountain AHEC

Ouimette, Ruth   FNP Program faculty; also, the first FNP to hold a graduate faculty appointment in the School of Nursing

Perry, Evelyn   Dean, East Carolina University School of Nursing

Pickard, Faye   Associate professor, UNC School of Nursing; worked in the UNC continuing care clinic

Pickard, Glenn	Medical director, Family Nurse Practitioner Program; faculty, UNC School of Medicine; considered the "founder" of North Carolina's FNP Program
Schafer, Donna	First FNP at Walstonburg Health Center, the first community clinic established by the North Carolina Office of Rural Health
Sheps, Cecil	Vice chancellor of health affairs, University of North Carolina at Chapel Hill
Solberg, Patricia	Lawyer with the Institute of Government, University of North Carolina at Chapel Hill; served as legal counsel and lobbyist for the North Carolina Nurses Association
Stead, Eugene**	Founder and first director of the Duke University Physician Assistant Program
Warren, David	Lawyer with the Institute of Government University of North Carolina at Chapel Hill; drafted the first piece of legislation enabling FNP and PA practice
Warren, Geneva	A Prospect Hill community activist who prodded UNC to provide health services in Prospect Hill; served as administrative assistant to Governor Jim Hunt's wife, Carolyn Hunt
Watkins, Judy (aka Julia)	Director of the UNC School of Nursing Family Nurse Practitioner Program
Wilkman, Margaret	One of the early FNP nurse faculty and one of the first FNPs to practice at the Prospect Hill clinic
Williams, Carolyn	Faculty, UNC School of Nursing; principal investigator of the FNP-PRIMEX program evaluation project
Wilson, Glenn	Founder and first director of the North Carolina AHEC Program, UNC School of Medicine
Wilson, Ruby	Faculty, Duke University School of Nursing; collaborator with Ingles and Stead in Duke nursing practice experiments

**Notes and/or letters rather than audiotapes.

Twelve Miles Up the Road: Duke University's Nursing Experiments and PA Program

Invariably, in many of the early discussions about the nurse practitioner movement in North Carolina, comparisons were made between the Physician Assistant (PA) Program at Duke University, twelve miles up the road from the University of North Carolina (UNC), and the Family Nurse Practitioner Program at UNC. Such comparisons were inevitable as the Duke PA Program began in the mid-sixties, around the same time that UNC was contemplating the value of a nurse practitioner role in its own continuing care experiments.[1] And certainly, the "FNP at UNC" and the "PA at Duke" crisscrossed often as these new programs were discussed by nurses and physicians across the state. This was especially true when the question of legal authorization was addressed, particularly since the public saw no clear or obvious distinctions between NPs and PAs.

The purpose here is not to recap the history of the PA development. However, there were clinical and educational nursing trials at Duke University that preceded the PA Program. These experiments are related in some ways to North Carolina's nurse practitioner movement, and to nursing practice in general. The nurse practitioner experiments at UNC sought an innovation or advancement in clinical nursing practice. The nursing experiments at Duke during the 1950s likewise represented early innovative thinking about the clinical roles and education of nurses. No matter how innovative, they both were resisted and shaped by the profession's accepted way of thinking and doing—the conventional wisdom at the time.

Although unintended, a profession's certifying bodies and regulatory authorities often limit innovative thinking and experimentation. However, UNC's Family Nurse Practitioner Program, like other early nurse practitioner programs, found ways to work around the restrictive bonds of their professional associations. Unfortunately, the nursing experiments conducted at Duke University did not—and thus, Duke University choose the physician assistant route.

THE CLINICAL AND EDUCATIONAL NURSING TRIALS AT DUKE

In the 1950s, several influential Duke nurses and physicians were interested in demonstrating ways for nurses to assume greater patient care responsibility as well as strengthen the collaborative relationship between doctors and nurses. In Duke's newly revised BSN program, nursing faculty were committed to flexibility and independent study within the curriculum. Senior students selected a clinical area for a focused experience and were encouraged to work closely with physicians and other clinical providers in their chosen clinical area to expand and deepen their knowledge and abilities.

In 1956, Duke offered a newly designed nursing master's program also based on the faculty's commitment to clinical excellence and nurse–physician collaboration. It differed significantly from the normative nursing master's programs offered at the time that emphasized the functional areas of teaching or administration. The "new" mid-1950s master's program started at Duke became the prevailing model twenty years later. But when first conceived, it was rejected outright by the profession. The School of Medicine at Duke was supportive of the nursing school's new direction. But since the School of Nursing could not go forward with its innovative master's program without accreditation, the School of Medicine moved in another direction and developed a physician assistant program.

The events at Duke during the 1950s and early 1960s provide additional insight into how organized nursing and medicine reacted to innovations at that time, and how they intersected with the nurse practitioner movement in North Carolina.

A Controversial Clinical Master's Program—Before Its Time

Thelma Ingles, professor and chair of medical–surgical nursing at Duke, was instrumental in establishing Duke's new four-year program leading to a Bachelor of Science in Nursing degree in 1953, as noted above.[2] Ingles, a pioneer always looking for new and better ways, then turned her attention to a master's degree program. Ingles believed that

> until we advanced their *nursing* knowledge and skills, nurses could never improve the profession—certainly they would not have the knowledge necessary for teaching and administration.[3]

She set out to develop a new master's program at Duke—one that would be nothing like the typical master's programs offered at the time, with their emphasis on administration or teaching. The course of study she envisioned was to prepare clinical practitioners, what we would describe today as "advanced" clinical practitioners.

Ingles knew what she wanted to accomplish with the new program, but as she reflected,

> it soon became clear to me that I was not prepared to teach these students, nor could I find anyone around the area who was capable. I decided I would have to go back to school. I visited almost all of the major university programs and found none that could meet

my needs. Almost all of them, master's programs, had a minimum number of hours of nursing.[4]

Not finding any established program that would meet her needs for advanced clinical knowledge, Ingles found an alternative: she spent a sabbatical year studying with Eugene Stead, Jr., MD, chair of the Department of Medicine at Duke. As Ingles describes this year of study,

> We had no model on which to plan such a year and no clear idea about how we would work, so we decided to begin and see what directions evolved. I made rounds with him and his interns and residents and periodically selected a patient for protracted study. I had regular conferences with Dr. Stead at which he would quiz me.[5]

She saw not only patients in the hospital but also met with family members and visited their homes.

At the end of her sabbatical year, Ingles felt she was an "educated nurse" with advanced clinical knowledge. She wanted to incorporate her learnings in a new master's program. Knowing they would need funds to start the program she envisioned, Ingles submitted a proposal to the Rockefeller Foundation to establish a new Master of Science in Nursing (MSN) program to prepare advanced clinical practitioners. Duke's program would require thirty units of nursing courses and twelve units in supporting arts and science courses, in contrast with other master's programs that offered only a few courses focusing on clinical nursing. Ingles submitted her proposal to the Rockefeller Foundation, and in early August 1957, the Rockefeller Foundation awarded Duke $250,000 for this clinical master's program. By the end of that August, Ingles had recruited five students to the first class.

The clinical master's program was controversial. It contrasted starkly with traditional graduate programs intended to prepare nurses for teaching or supervisory positions. When the National League for Nursing (NLN), the accrediting body for nursing, reviewed the program the first time, they declined to accredit it. It was just too great a change from the status quo. They did not see "advanced clinical education" as anything more than "a repetition of the basic program [for nurses],"[6] and it did not prepare students for teaching and administration—in their view, the prime purpose of a Master in Science in Nursing degree. They were suspicious of the close collaboration and involvement of physicians in the program, something that was to Ingles a premise for excellent clinical practice. Further, the NLN found Ingles inadequately prepared to direct this program. First, her advanced clinical knowledge came as a result of her sabbatical with Stead—a physician. Second, they found her only formal preparation in nursing at the diploma level to be inadequate to direct a master's program.

In response to the criticism about her preparation, Ingles took a leave and enrolled in the NLN-recommended "education" courses at the University of California, Berkeley—as Ingles says, "not for my sake, but for the accreditor's sake."[7] She continued, "When the NLN accreditors turned the program down the second time, I felt I had no choice but to resign [from the graduate program]. I couldn't let students invest a year's work in a program that was not accredited by the NLN."[8]

Ingles had taken a circuitous route into nursing: first, a BA from UCLA, then a diploma from Mass General Hospital, then an MA from Case Western Reserve University. She would add to those credentials her year of sabbatical study with Dr. Stead, what to her was one of the most valuable parts of her education. By this time, she was known as a national and international leader. Her ideas for nursing education and clinical practice were ahead of her time—perhaps too revolutionary, which was undoubtedly true of the clinical master's program she developed.

At the time, nursing associations, schools of nursing, and the profession rejected her ideas. Of course, the NLN's repudiation of the new program was a severe blow to Ingles. But as with many innovations initially cast aside, the good ones eventually become the conventional ones. Today, a clinical emphasis in graduate programs in nursing is the norm.

The Hanes Project: Demonstrating Innovative Clinical Practice

The "Hanes Project" was not a demonstration of the nurse practitioner role, but it had the potential to change the face of nursing practice in hospitals and beyond, and it also held the promise of changing the financing of nursing services. But its intention to "expand" the practice of nursing and elevate nurses' clinical work was highly percipient. It likely would have morphed into what we now know as nurse practitioner work or as advanced clinical practice.

Stead and Ingles had collaborated on the new master's curriculum, but since that initiative was rejected, they once again worked on designing a new nursing practice model—an all-RN staff. In their model, patients would be assigned to one of three levels of intensity of care for nursing services. Importantly, each level would be associated with a different charge for services. Stead had managed to convince hospital administrators to include a separate line item on the hospital bill for nursing services, the first time a hospital would bill separately for nursing services! These fees would be invested in the School of Nursing as highly educated faculty were an integral part of Hanes's nursing services.

Ruby Wilson returned to Duke after completing her master's degree and was involved in Duke's newly implemented baccalaureate program. When the 1961 BSN class graduated, they met informally among themselves. They then went to Ingles, the department head of medical–surgical nursing at the time and asked if there was "any way they could practice nursing the way that they had been taught, and that if they could, they would be willing to stay at Duke."[9] Ingles went to Wilson because Wilson had known these students-now-graduates as seniors. Wilson recalls that "the class that graduated in '61, I will never forget them because, to me, they were the most outstanding group of students that I had ever taught."[10] Ingles had another idea percolating in her head, and the class of '61 gave her the impetus to try something new again.

Ingles and Wilson discussed their ideas, and Ingles called on Stead with the concept she and Wilson had come up with, namely, to take a unit in the hospital and staff that unit with the BSN graduates of the class of '61. All the necessary hospital and school authorities approved the proposed project, and Wilson became coordinator of the "Hanes Project."

As Wilson notes, Ingles was great with ideas, but not so great with the practical implementation of those ideas.

> We worked well together because she would bring up some ideas, we would discuss them, but then it was up to me to implement them, and at the time she thought I was too pragmatic—but actually, somebody had to be pragmatic with Thelma.[11]

At this time, Ingles left for her sabbatical at the University of California, Berkeley while Wilson spent the summer working out the details.

Dr. Eugene Stead, Jr., the influential chair of medicine at Duke, convinced hospital officials to dedicate a ward for the nursing demonstration project. Stead had always been a staunch supporter of nurses, and his collaboration with nurses who exemplified a commitment to the highest level of clinical excellence buoyed his support. Stead also believed that nurses and doctors working together collaboratively provided better patient care than either one working on their own. Wilson was instrumental in selecting the demonstration unit. According to Wilson, they chose the Hanes unit for the project because the head nurse, Mrs.

Whitaker, supported the new baccalaureate program and would likely support the project. With hospital support, Wilson and Stead collaborating, and the unit selected, the Hanes Project began.

During the Hanes Project year, BSN graduates provided continuity of care to a set of thirty-five patients in a private medical clinical unit—the Hanes Ward, as it was named then. Wilson and the graduate nurses

> tested a variety of approaches to patient care, adopting those that proved successful. Each patient admitted to the ward was assigned a nurse as well as a physician. Both assessed the patient's needs. Nursing and medical orders were written side by side on the same page to improve communication with all caregivers. The patient–nurse–physician relationship was the focal point of the project, and soon staff physicians were asking to have their patients admitted to Hanes.[12]

The support of Stead was valuable to the success of the project. Wilson describes how she made rounds with Stead and the residents. Stead listened to Wilson's ideas and questions and even invited comments. Sometimes Stead would query Wilson first. Residents were initially stunned, but they soon learned that "whatever was going to happen on that ward was going to happen because I [Wilson] had Gene Stead's support."[13] And eventually, the residents learned to ask the nurses about their patients. Residents even came in ahead of rounds to talk with the nurses so they would be more fully informed when it came time to make rounds with Stead.

> To Wilson, the goal of the Hanes Project
> was to demonstrate that graduates of baccalaureate programs were indeed competent in clinical practice, given time for adjustment

to being a graduate nurse, but also given an environment condu-cive—a flexible environment.... We kept saying during the entire time that we were going to try different things.[14]

Later, nurses from across the country would tell Wilson that hers was the first primary nursing project in the country. Indeed, it was, although in 1961 the concept of "primary nursing" was not yet fully conceived.

By March 1962, Wilson had to decide whether to continue with some version of the nursing practice demonstration on Hanes. She had ideas about including more units and linking the practice demonstration with both baccalaureate and graduate students. She knew they needed more nurses to staff these units, but by March, it was too late to recruit the numbers of nurses required. The Hanes Project lasted only a year, but not without long-lasting effects. Influential physicians were impressed. Wilson said twenty years later:

And even today I'll see Dr. [Edward S.] Orgain, and a number of those, and they'll say, "That was the best nursing care, and I will say the best patient care altogether that we ever gave in this hospital, because of the working together of physicians and nurses." And for a long time, he kept saying, "When are we going to have another Hanes Project?"[15]

Everyone associated with the Hanes Project was disappointed it would not continue, but the faculty and financial resources needed to continue were not available. Ingles had already left Duke after the master's program was denied accreditation on its second review. Ruby Wilson was conflicted about ending the Hanes Project, but she had an opportunity to develop another innovation at Duke. A new type of nursing position was created on the nephrology unit, the first clinical specialist position at Duke University.

Wilson took this position and held it for several years while advocating for more nurse clinical specialists' positions at the Duke University Hospital. Stead, disappointed as well, turned his attention elsewhere.

THE PHYSICIAN ASSISTANT (PA) PROGRAM: "FROM THOSE ASHES"

Stead had been a champion of nurses throughout his early medical career. He felt they were underutilized and capable of much more than they were allowed by law or convention. Stead himself said he had opposed the idea of training corpsmen as physician assistants, but admittedly, he had no rationale for his opposition. Initially, he wholeheartedly joined with nursing in moving toward an advanced clinical role for nurses. Harvey Estes, a colleague of Stead's, thought that Stead was enthusiastic about the nursing experiments he was involved with and supported. But the NLN rejection embittered him and turned him away from nursing. As Estes described it, it was "from those ashes" that the PA Program came to be.[16] After the second NLN rejection of the clinical nursing master's program, Stead retreated from the nursing experiment and the Hanes Project.

By his accounting, Stead was unaware of other expanded nursing role experiments taking place across the country, including the emerging thinking about nurse practitioners just twelve miles down the road at UNC. But after the rebuff of Duke's master's program by the NLN, Stead took notice of other experiments using ex-military corpsmen; he was also influenced by what his good friend Amos Johnson had been doing in his private practice in Garland, North Carolina.

Johnson, a physician practicing in rural eastern North Carolina, was interested in being involved with the professional medical societies. Many solo physicians in private practice were tied to their practice obligations, requiring them to limit their involvement in professional society activities. Johnson was one of these at first, but soon he discovered he needed assistants—and saw that the best way to get assistants was to train them himself.

In the 1940s, Johnson recruited a young African American, Henry "Buddy" Treadwell, to work in his office as an orderly. Gradually, Johnson taught Treadwell to do more in his practice. Soon, Treadwell was viewed as Johnson's assistant. For twenty-seven years, Johnson and Treadwell worked as a team, and Treadwell functioned as a PA—long before the term had been coined. In a feature article in the May 1967 issue of *Medical Economics* describing the working relationship between the two, Johnson said: "Treadwell works for me much as a resident in a hospital works for an attending."[17] Knowing firsthand the work of Johnson and Treadwell, Stead began plans to recruit corpsmen for a new training program, thankful he would not have any nursing accrediting bodies overseeing his new program.

In 1967, as the first graduates of the PA Program were ready to enter the field, Stead and other faculty began to think about the legal status of PAs. As described in chapter 8, Duke hosted four national conferences on PA education and legal/ethical issues. The legal model adopted by North Carolina was set in those early conferences sponsored by Duke. PA practice was legitimized as an exception to the Medical Practice Act. The Board of Medicine would write rules governing PA practice and would be the body granting practice approval to individual PAs.

Several years later, the issue of NP legal recognition in North Carolina was discussed. Governmental authorities and regulatory bodies, along with many physicians and nurses, could not fathom any form of "enabling legislation," as it was called, other than to model NP legislation after the PA legislation. The mold was cast. From a legal standpoint, little distinction was made between the two providers. And from those early years on to this day, North Carolina continues to be one of the states with the most restrictive NP enabling legislation—all of which is discussed in chapter 8 and chapter 11.

Lists of Acronyms and Figures

ACRONYMS

ACRONYM	FULL NAME
AACN	American Association of Colleges of Nursing
ADN	Associate Degree in Nursing
AHEC	Area Health Education Center
AMA	American Medical Association
ANA	American Nurses Association
APN/APRN	Advanced Practice Nurse/Advanced Practice Registered Nurse
BSN	Bachelor of Science in Nursing Degree
CAA	Community Action Agency—a local program office of the U.S. Government Office of Economic Opportunity
CAP	Community Action Program
CCU	Coronary Care Unit
CE	Continuing Education
DBA	Doctor of Business Administration Degree
DHEW	Department of Health, Education, and Welfare
DNP	Doctor of Nursing Practice Degree
DPH	Doctor of Public Health Degree
Duke	Duke University—Durham, North Carolina
EAHEC	Eastern Area Health Education Center
ECU	East Carolina University—Greenville, North Carolina
FDR	Franklin Delano Roosevelt
FNP/FNPs	Family Nurse Practitioner(s)
FNS	Frontier Nursing Service
HSRC	Health Services Research Center
ICU/CCU	Intensive Care Unit/Critical Care Unit/Coronary Care Unit
MAHEC	Mountain Area Health Education Center
MBA	Master of Business Administration Degree

MD	Doctor of Medicine Degree
MPH	Master of Public Health Degree
MSN	Master of Science in Nursing Degree
NCAT	North Carolina Agricultural and Technical State University
NCBM	North Carolina Board of Medicine
NCBN	North Carolina Board of Nursing
NCHSRD	National Center for Health Services Research and Development
NCJPC	North Carolina Joint Practice Commission
NCMS	North Carolina Medical Society
NCNA	North Carolina Nurses Association
NJPC	National Joint Practice Committee
NLN	National League for Nursing
NP/NPs	Nurse Practitioner(s)—used generically to include all nurse practitioners in contrast with "family" nurse practitioners, "pediatric" nurse practitioners, et al.
OCCHS	Orange–Chatham Comprehensive Health Service
OEO	Office of Economic Opportunity
PA/PAs	Physician Assistant(s)
PhD	Doctor of Philosophy Degree
PNP/PNPs	Pediatric Nurse Practitioner(s)
PRIMEX	Primary Care Extenders
RMP/NCRMP	Regional Medical Program/North Carolina Regional Medical Program
RN	Registered Nurse
SON	School of Nursing
SPH	School of Public Health
UN	United Nations
UNC/UNC-CH	University of North Carolina at Chapel Hill
WAHEC	Wilmington Area Health Education Center
WCU	Western Carolina University—Cullowhee, North Carolina
WIC	Women, Infants, and Children—a federal program providing grants to states for supplemental nutrition assistance for low-income pregnant and postpartum women and children under five years of age

FIGURES

ENDNOTES

CHAPTER ONE

1 Gale Adcock, "Advocate Like a Nurse," *Tar Heel Nurse: Special 2021 Legislative Issue* 83, no. 2 (Winter 2021): 13.

2 Traditional narrative is used here to distinguish it from modern narrative. Traditional narrative focuses on the chronology of events, and individuals and their intentions, while modern narrative focuses on concepts and trends. Traditional narrative allows the author to tell a story, and via the story, provide interpretation and analysis.

3 Alfred Yankauer and Judith Sullivan, "The New Health Professionals: Three Examples," *Annual Review of Public Health*, no. 3 (1982): 252.

4 Julie Fairman, *Making Room in the Clinic: Nurse Practitioners and the Evolution of Modern Health Care* (New Brunswick, NJ: Rutgers University Press, 2008), 2.

5 Appendix A provides details about the *Conversations Collection*, part of the Cynthia M. Freund Papers, Barbara Bates Center for the Study of the History of Nursing, University of Pennsylvania. Quotations and summaries from the Conversations Collection are used throughout the book and follow the *Chicago Manual of Style* guidelines for unpublished conversation and interview notes, such as John Doe in discussion with the author and Booth, date, page number, Freund Papers, Univ. of Penn. Subsequent shortened notes follow a similar form, such as John Doe, discussion, date, page number.

CHAPTER TWO

1 Betty Compton in discussion with the author and Booth, June 2, 1982, 5, Freund Papers, Univ. of Penn.

2 Leonard I. Stein, "The Doctor-Nurse Game," *American Journal of Nursing* 16, no. 6 (1967): 101–05; and Barbara Bates, "Doctor and Nurse: Changing Roles and Relations," *New England Journal of Medicine*, no. 283 (July 16, 1970): 129–34.

3 James A. Bryan, William W. McLendon, and Katherine Savage, *Medicine at Chapel Hill: The Department of Medicine at the University of North Carolina 1952–2007* (Chapel Hill: The Department of Medicine, School of Medicine, The University of North Carolina at Chapel Hill, 2012), 159–61.

4 Lucy Conant handwritten letter to Audrey Booth, stamped February 1, 1983, Freund Papers, Univ. of Penn.

5 Conant, letter, February 1, 1983, 1.

6 Harvey L. Smith. *A Community's View of Health Care: The Prospect Hill Study* (Chapel Hill: Division of Health Affairs, University of North Carolina at Chapel Hill, 1970).

7 "History of the Community Action Program Office," National Archives, Records of the Community Services Administration, www.archives.gov/research/guide-fed-records/groups/381.html#381.3.12 .

8   Frank Conant, "Lucy H. Conant: Her Two Lives," unpublished book, Freund Papers, Univ. of Penn., 15.

9   Conant, "Lucy H. Conant: Her Two Lives," 35.

10 Conant, "Lucy H. Conant: Her Two Lives," 49.

11 Conant, "Lucy H. Conant: Her Two Lives," 51.

12 Conant, "Lucy H. Conant: Her Two Lives," 45.

CHAPTER THREE

1   The author acknowledges that the terms "doctor" or "doctors" can reference those who hold doctoral degrees other than the MD (Doctor of Medicine) degree, such as the PhD, DBA, DNP, DPH, etc. However, using the term "physician(s)" to refer to MDs in all instances can result in an overly repetitive and cumbersome read. Therefore, throughout the book, the terms "doctor(s)" and "physician(s)" will be used interchangeably when the context clearly indicates that "doctor(s)" refer specifically to medical doctors. When the context is broad or nonspecific, the term "physician(s)" will be used when referring to those holding the Doctor of Medicine degree.

2   Franklin Delano Roosevelt (FDR) had included the right to health care in his proposed Second Bill of Rights, which was never adopted before of his death. Eleanor Roosevelt, however, took his work to the United Nations (UN), where it was codified and adopted by all nations of the UN, including the United States. Twenty-plus years later, Dr. Martin Luther King, Jr., again pushed for a declaration of health care as a right in the United States, but the Civil Rights Act of 1964 did not guarantee health care as a right. Another forty-five years later, President Obama in commenting on the passage of the Affordable Care Act, declared health care a right for all Americans. However, others point out a significant difference between declaring health care a right and the guarantee and provision of health care for all as a right. For differing discussions on "health care as a right," see Mary Gerish, "Health Care as a Human Right," "The State of Healthcare in the United States," special issue, in *Human Rights Magazine* 43, no. 3, www.americanbar.org/groups/crsj/publications/human_rights_magazine_home/the-state-of-healthcare-in-the-united-states/health-care-as-a-human-right/; Vann R. Newkirk II, "The Fight for Health Care Has Always Been about Civil Rights," *The Atlantic*, June 27, 2017, www.theatlantic.com/politics/archive/2017/06/the-fight-for-health-care-is-really-all-about-civil-rights/531855/; and Mahiben Maruthappu, Rele Ologunde, and Ayinkeran Gunarajasingam, "Is Health Care a Right? Health Reforms in the USA and Their Impact upon the Concept of Care," *Annals of Medicine and Surgery (London)* 2, no. 1 (2013): 15–17, doi:10.1016/S2049-0801(13)70021-9, www.ncbi.nlm.nih.gov/pmc/articles/PMC4326121/.

3   See T. Elaine Adamson, "Critical Issues in the Use of Physician Associates and Assistants," *American Journal of Public Health* 61, no. 9 (September 1971): 1765–79; Charles Lewis and Barbara Resnick, "Nurse Clinics and Progressive Ambulatory Patient Care," *New England Journal of Medicine* 277, no. 23 (December 1967): 1236–1241; John W. Runyan, Jr., William E. Phillips, and Odie Herring, "A Program for the Care of Patients with Chronic Diseases," *JAMA* 211, no. 3 (January 1970): 476–81; Loretta C. Ford and Henry K. Silver, "The Expanded Role of the Nurse in Child Care," *Nursing Outlook* XV (September 1967): 33–45.

4   American Medical Association, *Directory of Approved Internships and Residencies 1967–1968* (Chicago: AMA, 1967), 6.

5   Board of Governors, University of North Carolina, *Special Committee to Study the Request of East Carolina University for a Second Year of Medical Education, December 29, 1972* (Chapel Hill: Board of Governors, University of North Carolina, 1972). The report documented the maldistribution of physicians across North Carolina.

6   Ad Hoc Committee of Health Professions, *Extending the Scope of Nursing Practice* (Washington: U.S. Government Printing Office, 1972), 2.

7   See appendix B for a fuller discussion of the nursing experiments at Duke University.

8   Glenn Pickard in discussion with the author and Booth, August 1982, tape 1, 55, Freund Papers, Univ. of Penn.

9   "Twentieth-Century North Carolina Timeline," North Carolina Museum of History, www.ncmuseumofhistory.org/learning/educators/timelines/twentieth-century-north-carolina-timeline; Helen Thomas, "It's All Up to You! North Carolina and the Good Health Program, Part I," *Southern Sources: Exploring the Southern History Collection* (blog), May 6, 2014, blogs.lib.unc.edu/shc/2014/05/06/its-all-up-to-you-north-carolina-and-the-good-health-program-part-1/.

10   Governor's Commission on State Hospital and Medical Care, To All the People of North Carolina: A Proposed State-wide Program of Hospital and Medical Care, presented to the Joint Session of the North Carolina House and Senate. The Medical Care Commission Act was ratified on March 21, 1945 (NCGS 143B-165). www.ncleg.net/EnactedLegislation/Statutes/HTML/BySection/Chapter_143B/GS_143B-165.html.

11   Glenn Pickard, August 1982, tape 1, 2.

12   A fuller discussion of the contributions of the early physicians recruited to the Department of Medicine can be found in James A. Bryan II, William W. McLendon, and Katherine D. Savage, *Medicine at Chapel Hill: The Department of Medicine at the University of North Carolina 1952–2007* (Chapel Hill: The Department of Medicine, School of Medicine, The University of North Carolina at Chapel Hill, 2012).

13   Kerr L. White, R. Franklin Williams, and Bernard G. Greenberg, "The Ecology of Medical Care," *New England Journal of Medicine* 265 (November 2, 1961): 885–92.

14   Glenn Pickard, August 1982, tape 1, 3.

15   Glenn Pickard, August 1982, tape 1, 4–5.

16   Some of the nurses in the general clinic and continuing care clinic were Betty West, Judy (Julia Day) Watkins, and Mary Cochran. Watkins would later become codirector of the UNC Nurse Practitioner Program.

17   In the mid-sixties, Chatham County was a small rural county immediately south of the UNC Medical Center.

18   For an extensive discussion of the many phases of the "continuing care clinic" demonstration, see Bryan, McLendon, and Savage, *Medicine at Chapel Hill*, 59, 62, and 158–59.

19   Ford and Silver, "The Expanded Role of the Nurse in Child Care," 33–45; and Charles E. Lewis and Barbara A. Resnick, "Activities, Events and Outcomes in Ambulatory Patient Care," *New England Journal of Medicine* CCXXC (March 20, 1969): 645–49.

20   M. Virginia Dryden, *Nursing Trends* (Dubuque, IA: Wm. C. Brown Company, 1968);

Carolyn R. Aradine and Marc C. Hansen, "Nursing in a Primary Care Setting," *Nursing Outlook* XVIII (April 1970): 45–46; Ethel Gozzi, Glen Austin, and Alfred Yankauer, "Pediatric Nurse Practitioner at Work," American Journal of Nursing, no. 11 (November 1970): 2372–74; and Eloise P. Lewis, ed., *Changing Patterns of Nursing Practice: New Needs, New Roles* (New York: The American Journal of Nursing Company, 1971).

CHAPTER FOUR

1 Harvey L. Smith, *A Community's View of Health Care: The Prospect Hill Study* (Chapel Hill: Division of Health Affairs, University of North Carolina at Chapel Hill, 1970), 11.

2 Mrs. Joseph H., "Lifetime of Medical Practice to Be Climaxed with the Building of Clinic," *Caswell County Messenger* (Yanceyville, North Carolina), May 16, 1957, 1, 5.

3 A chart displaying the genealogical lines of the influential Scotts discussed here is appended at the end of the chapter. This information is adapted from "The Scott Family Collection: Family Tree," http://www.scottcollection.org/family-tree/.

4 Geneva Warren in discussion with the author and Booth, September 26, 1982, 3, Freund Papers, Univ. of Penn.

5 The above transactions are documented in a series of letters sent to and from Geneva Warren. Copies of the letters can be found in "Letters: Geneva Warren," the *Conversations Collection*, Freund Papers, Univ. of Penn.

6 Geneva Warren, September 26, 1982, 4.

7 Robert E. Ireland, "Institute of Government," January 2006, www.ncpedia.org/institute-government.

8 David Warren in discussion with the author and Booth, September 28, 1982, 20, Freund Papers, Univ. of Penn.

9 Cecil Sheps in discussion with the author and Booth, June 1, 1981, 1, Freund Papers, Univ. of Penn.

10 Cecil Sheps, discussion, June 1, 1981, 1.

11 Loretta C. Ford and Henry K. Silver, "The Expanded Role of the Nurse in Child Care," *Nursing Outlook* XV (September 1967): 33–45.

12 Cecil Sheps, discussion, June 1, 1981, 2.

13 The University of Michigan, Ann Arbor.

14 Donald L. Madison, "The Work of James D. Bernstein of North Carolina," *North Carolina Medical Journal* 67, no. 1 (January 2012): 28.

15 James Bernstein in discussion with the author and Booth, August 25, 1982, 1–2, Freund Papers, Univ. of Penn.

16 James Bernstein, discussion, August 25, 1982, 2.

17 A North Carolina Foundation dedicated to improving the lives of all North Carolinians.

18 Cecil Sheps, discussion, June 1, 1981, 13.

19 Linda Mashburn in discussion with the author and Booth, September 27, 1982, 1, Freund Papers, Univ. of Penn.

20 Linda Mashburn, discussion, September 27, 1982, 6.

21 Linda Mashburn, discussion, September 27, 1982, 7.

22 Linda Mashburn, discussion, September 27, 1982, 19. The foundation Mashburn references

was the Appalachian Commission Fund, which she clarified in a March 24, 2021, email to the author, Freund Papers, Univ. of Penn.

23 Linda Mashburn, discussion, September 27, 1982, 5.

24 Confirmed by Mashburn in a March 24, 2021 email, Freund Papers, Univ. of Penn.

25 Geneva Warren, September 26, 1982, 16.

26 The university's name from 1932 to 1963. After that and until the present, it has been referred to as the University of North Carolina at Greensboro.

27 Geneva Warren, discussion, September 26, 1982, 2.

28 Geneva Warren, discussion, September 26, 1982, 9.

29 Gordon H. DeFriese, "Cecil G. Sheps," *Encyclopedia Britannica*, February 4, 2021, www.britannica.com/biography/Cecil-G-Sheps.

30 Donald L. Madison, "Remembering Cecil," *North Carolina Medical Journal* 65, no. 5 (September–October 2004): 301–06.

31 Donald L. Madison, "The Work of James D. Bernstein," *North Carolina Medical Journal* 67, no. 1 (January/February 2006): 27–42.

CHAPTER FIVE

1 Julia (Judy) Watkins, a very supportive School of Public Health faculty member, joined the School of Nursing faculty as associate director of the FNP Program in 1970 and became its codirector in 1972, serving in that capacity through 1978 when the certificate program merged into the nursing school's master's degree program.

2 Glenn Pickard, discussion, August 26, 1982, 1–2.

3 Glenn Pickard, discussion, August 26, 1982, 14.

4 William Fleming, Bernard Greenberg, Robert Huntley, Kerr White, and T. Franklin Williams.

5 Carolyn Williams in discussion with the author and Booth, June 1, 1982, 10, Freund Papers, Univ. of Penn.

6 Carolyn Williams, discussion, June 1, 1982, 6.

7 Medical and public health faculty working to develop new primary care systems at UNC.

8 Faye Pickard in discussion with the author and Booth, September 28, 1982, 3, Freund Papers, Univ. of Penn.

9 Mary Gwen (Pickard) Phillips, written personal note to the author, February 26, 2021, Freund Papers, Univ. of Penn.

10 Amie Modigh, personal discussion with the author, in or around 1978.

11 The recruitment of a black faculty member was a crucial first step in changing the image of the school held by nurses of color in North Carolina. The SON admitted its first students in 1950 but did not admit its first students of color until 1963, when three black students were admitted to the master's program. The first black student was admitted to the undergraduate program in 1965. Black nurses were embittered by the school's admission policies; some had received letters flatly stating that black students were not eligible for admission to the school. Their justifiable anger persisted into the nineties, even though black students had been admitted in increasing numbers since the mid-sixties.

12 Julie Fairman and Joan Lynaugh, *Critical Care Nursing: A History* (Philadelphia: University of Pennsylvania Press, 1998).

13 W. Bruce Fye, "Resuscitating a Circulation Abstract to Celebrate the 50th Anniversary of the Coronary Care Unit Concept," *Circulation* 124, no. 17 (2011): 1886.

14 Roland H. Berg, "More than a Nurse, Less than a Doctor," *Look Magazine*, September 6, 1966, 57–59, 61.

15 For an excellent discussion of the ANA–AMA exchanges during this period, see Natalie Holt, "'Confusion's Masterpiece': The Development of the Physician Assistant Profession," *Bulletin of the History of Medicine* 72, no. 2 (1998): 246–78.

16 This definition contains a slight modification made in 1975, when the original was reviewed by the Family Nurse Practitioner Faculty Consortium, which included the Schools of Nursing at East Carolina University and the University of North Carolina at Chapel Hill, and the FNP Program offered by the Mountain AHEC, with academic certification from UNC.

17 Julia Watkins in discussion with the author and Booth, November 9, 1982, 2, Freund Papers, Univ. of Penn.

18 Betty Sue Johnson, in discussion with the author and Booth, September 2, 1982, 15, Freund Papers, Univ. of Penn.

19 Betty Sue Johnson, discussion, September 2, 1982, 20.

20 In retrospect, nurse practitioner opponents and proponents were not that far apart. Johnson recalled working on an early curriculum committee in 1966 and 1967, initiated by nurse faculty from the School of Public Health. Betty Sue Johnson had submitted recommendations about nurse practitioner training, which had been incorporated in the minutes. As she was preparing to leave the School of Nursing in 1978, she received a note from Glenn Pickard with a copy of her recommendations. He said: "Betty Sue, I've just been going through some of the old files of the nurse practitioner movement. Your recommendations, almost to the letter, describe what we wanted this program to be." Glenn Pickard, discussion, September 28, 1982, 32.

21 Conant, letter, February 1, 1983, 2.

22 Faye Pickard, discussion, September 28, 1982, 11.

23 The actual timing was in spring 1970.

24 Judy Watkins, discussion, November 9, 1982, 3.

25 Judy Watkins, discussion, November 9, 1982, 3.

26 An interim budget process allowing for additional budget requests to be considered by the state legislature.

27 Glenn Pickard, discussion, August 26, 1982, 23–24.

28 Glenn Pickard, discussion, August 26, 1982, 26.

29 Glenn Pickard, discussion, August 26, 1982, 26.

30 Glenn Pickard, discussion, August 26, 1982, 27.

31 Glenn Pickard, discussion, August 26, 1982, 28.

32 Glenn Pickard, discussion, August 26, 1982, 17.

33 Conant, letter, February 1, 1983, 1–2.

34 Glenn Pickard, discussion, September 1982, 20.

35 Glenn Pickard, discussion, September 1982, 20.

36 "Eulogy: Audrey Booth," the *Conversations Collection*, Freund Papers, Univ. of Penn.

CHAPTER SIX

1   Jean Dowdy, Marjorie Land, and Hargraves, Glenda, eds., *Reflections of Rural Health in Piedmont, North Carolina* (Sanford, NC: Triple J Publishing, LLC, 2015), 9.

2   "About Us: Piedmont Health Services," www.piedmonthealth.org/about-us/.

3   Jerry L. Weston, "Nurse Practitioners and Physician Assistants," in *Health United States, with Prevention Profile*, Department of Health and Human Services Publication No. (PHS) 81-1939 (Washington, D.C.: U.S. Government Printing Office, December 1980), 83.

4   Carolyn Williams, discussion, June 1, 1982.

5   See Madeline Leininger, D. Carnevali, and D. Little, "PRIMEX," *American Journal of Nursing* 72, no. 7 (July 1972).

6   See *PRIMEX CONSORTIUM*, Protocol for Health Services and Educational Evaluation Research, 1, Freund Papers, Univ. of Penn.

7   After 1971, provisions were made in the Nurse Training Act of 1971 (Public Law 92-158) for the training of nurse practitioners, administered by the Division of Nursing. See Weston, "Nurse Practitioners and Physician Assistants," 83.

8   Marie McIntyre was the first nurse codirector of the FNP Program, serving for two years in that capacity. Originally from the School of Public Health nursing faculty, she also held a joint faculty appointment in the School of Nursing.

9   Glenn Pickard, discussion, August 26, 1982, 30.

10 Ruth Efird, email message to the author, May 19, 2020, Freund Papers, Univ. of Penn.

11 Betty Compton, discussion, June 2, 1982, 2–3.

12 Institute of Medicine (U.S.), Division of Health Care Services, *Nursing and Nursing Education: Public Policies and Private Actions* (Washington, D.C.: National Academies Press, 1983), chapter 2.

13 Institute of Medicine (U.S.), Division of Health Care Services, *Report on the Shortages of Nurses and Other Medical Personnel in North Carolina, Report Number 10* (Raleigh, NC: North Carolina Legislative Research Commission, 1967), 63 and 105.

14 Interestingly, the 1967 legislative study commission referenced above was most concerned with the shortage of nurses, both practicing nurses and nursing faculty. They knew that baccalaureate programs were requisite to preparing teachers. Thus, they concluded that diploma nursing programs should be supported with state funds to continue increasing the supply of practicing nurses. The commission's recommendations received support from leading notables in nursing and medicine at the time, such as Margaret Dolan, chairman, legislative committee, North Carolina State Nurses Association; Edgar T. Beddingfield, chairman, legislative committee, Medical Society of North Carolina; Elizabeth S. Holley, chief, Public Health Nursing Section, North Carolina Board of Health; Marion Foster, executive director, North Carolina Hospital Association; and representatives of other professional associations.

15 Working paper, *Core Objectives for PRIMEX Programs: Conceptual Framework*, submitted by Eleanor C. Lambertsen of Cornell University–New York Hospital School of Nursing, April 24, 1973, to the Consortium for Evaluation of PRIMEX Programs, Freund Papers, Univ. of Penn.

16 Glenn Pickard, discussion, August 26, 1982, 40.

17 Margaret Wilkman in discussion with the author and Booth, December 16, 1982, 2–3, Freund Papers, Univ. of Penn.

18 Glenn Pickard, discussion, August 26, 1982, 29.

19 Margaret Wilkman, discussion, December 16, 1982, 3.

20 Margaret Wilkman, discussion, December 16, 1982, 4.

21 Margaret Wilkman, discussion, December 16, 1982, 4–5.

22 Betty Compton, discussion, June 2, 1982, 4–5.

23 Bob Lawrence, "Reflections on the Orange–Chatham Comprehensive Health Care Project," in *Reflections of Rural Health in Piedmont North Carolina*, eds. Jean Sandford Dowdy, Marjorie Land, and Glenda Hargraves (Sanford, NC: Triple J Publishing, LLC, 2015), 31.

24 Ruth Efird, email message to author, May 16, 2020.

25 Axalla Hoole, Robert Greenberg, and C. Glenn Pickard, "Acknowledgments," in *Patient Care Guidelines for Family Nurse Practitioners* (Little, Brown, and Company: Boston, 1976), xi.

26 Glenn Pickard, discussion, August 26, 1982, 39–40.

27 David Warren was, at the time, an attorney with UNC's Institute of Government; he worked with FNP faculty and supporters in examining the appropriate legal mechanisms to legitimize FNP practice.

28 Glenn Pickard, discussion, August 26, 1982, 40.

29 Glenn Pickard, discussion, August 26, 1982, 53.

30 Glenn Pickard, discussion, August 26, 1982, 54–55.

31 Margaret Wilkman, discussion, December 16, 1982, 8.

32 Geneva Warren, discussion, September 26, 1982, 12.

33 Glenn Pickard, discussion, August 26, 1982, 55–56.

34 Betty Compton, discussion, June 2, 1982, 11.

35 Betty Compton, phone conversation, May 20–25, 2020, wanting to make sure the record was correct.

CHAPTER SEVEN

1 OCCHS-sponsored students were Loretta Jean Dowdy, Glenda Hargraves, Lois Isler, Marjorie Land, and Hettie Garland, from Program Records, Freund Papers, Univ. of Penn.

2 Wake Memorial Hospital sponsored students were Norma Anderson, Elizabeth Brothers, and Ruth DeBrunner, from Program Records, Freund Papers, Univ. of Penn.

3 The Mt. Airy Private Practice–sponsored student was Dee Everhart. The Western Carolina Center–sponsored student was Mary Franklin. And the Pinehurst Medical Clinic–sponsored students were Nancy Kiser and Betty Yarborough. From Program Records, Freund Papers, Univ. of Penn.

4 Marjorie Land, in *Reflections of Rural Health in Piedmont North Carolina*, eds. Jean Dowdy, Marjorie Land, and Glenda Hargraves (Sandford, NC: Triple J Publishing, LLC, 2015), 61.

5 Glenda Oldham Hargraves, 'Time Well Spent," in *Reflections of Rural Health in Piedmont North Carolina*, 57.

6 Hargraves, "Time Well Spent," 57.

7   Agnes Binder-Weisiger, in discussion with the author, April 28, 2015, 2, Freund Papers, Univ. of Penn.

8   Cynthia M. Freund, "A Description of Family Nurse Practitioners' Activities" (master's thesis, School of Nursing, University of North Carolina at Chapel Hill, 1973).

9   Patricia Merwin, "An Analysis of Family Nurse Practitioner-Physician Consultations" (master's thesis, School of Nursing, University of North Carolina at Chapel Hill, 1977).

10 Michael J. Yedidia, *Delivering Primary Health Care: Nurse Practitioners at Work* (Boston: Auburn House Publishing Company, 1981), 21.

11 Donna Schafer in discussion with the author and Booth, Fall, 1982, 1, Freund Papers, Univ. of Penn.

12 Donna Schafer, discussion, Fall, 1982, 2.

13 Linda Mashburn, discussion, September 27, 1982, 8.

14 Glenn Wilson, "The Creation of the NC AHEC Program," in *North Carolina AHEC: Creating a Better State of Health for 40 Years* (Chapel Hill: University of North Carolina at Chapel Hill, June 6, 2012), 3.

15 Glenn Wilson in second discussion with the author, September 9, 1999, 23, Freund Papers, Univ. of Penn.

16 Faye Pickard, discussion, September 28, 1982, 5.

17 Wilson, "The Creation of the NC AHEC Program," 3.

18 James Bernstein, discussion, September 28, 1982, 4.

19 Cecil Sheps, discussion, June 1, 1982, 3.

20 Glenn Wilson, discussion, September 27, 1982, 7–8.

21 Glenn Wilson, discussion, September 27, 1982, 10.

22 Cecil Sheps, discussion, June 1, 1982, 4.

23 Glenn Wilson, discussion, September 27, 1982, 13.

24 James Holshouser in discussion with the author and Booth, August 25, 1982, 2, Freund Papers, Univ. of Penn.

25 James Holshouser, discussion, August 25, 1982, 2.

CHAPTER EIGHT

1   Faye Pickard, discussion, September 28, 1982, 8.

2   Evelyn Perry, personal communication, August 25, 1982, 20, Freund Papers, Univ. of Penn.

3   Evelyn Perry, personal communication, August 25, 1982, 25.

4   Evelyn Perry, personal communication, August 25, 1982, 25.

5   Mallie Penry was new to the ECU School of Nursing faculty, and although not prepared as a nurse practitioner, she was a public health nurse and very supportive of nurse practitioners.

6   Terry Lawler in discussion with the author, August 25, 1982, 21, Freund Papers, Univ. of Penn.

7   Evelyn Perry, personal communication, August 25, 1982, 22.

8   Freund Papers related to the Nurse Practitioner Movement: The Consortium of Statewide Nurse Practitioner Programs. See also "ECU-UNC FNP Meeting, October 18, 1974," Summary (aka Minutes), Freund Papers, Univ. of Penn.

9   Allison Armstrong was the first nurse practitioner, a PNP, appointed to the ECU School of Nursing faculty. Here Lawler is reflecting on the general faculty's view and opposition to nurse practitioners in describing how Armstrong was accepted by other faculty.

10   Terry Lawler, discussion, August 25, 1982, 14–15.

11   Evelyn Perry, personal communication, August 25, 1982, 15.

12   Martha Rogers, from New York University, was a nursing theoretician with a large following of those who had studied with her. She attempted to distinguish nursing from doctoring by emphasizing nursing theory and nursing diagnosis. She was very outspoken in opposition to nurse practitioners.

13   Katherine (Kit) Nuckolls in discussion with the author and Booth, August 24, 1982, 2, Freund Papers, Univ. of Penn.

14   Hettie Garland in discussion with the author and Booth, August 25, 1982, 10, Freund Papers, Univ. of Penn.

15   Hettie Garland, discussion, August 25, 1982, 10.

16   Laurel Copp had come as dean to the UNC School of Nursing in the summer of 1975.

17   Laurel Copp in discussion with Booth, September 3, 1982, 25, Freund Papers, Univ. of Penn.

18   Program Records, 1970–78, and various program reports, Freund Papers, Univ. of Penn.

19   "Appendix LP-1: Instructions for Logic Problems," *Terminal Progress Report on the Family Nurse Practitioner in North Carolina—PRIMEX, Grant No. HS 01333-03*, submitted to the Department of Health, Education, and Welfare, Health Resources Administration National Center for Health Services Research, by the University of North Carolina at Chapel Hill School of Nursing, June 1977, 1, Freund Papers, Univ. of Penn.

20   Logic Problems, *PRIMEX Grant*, 1–4.

21   Laurel Copp, discussion, September 3, 1982, 25.

CHAPTER NINE

1   U.S. Department of Health, Education, and Welfare, Report of the Surgeon General's Consultant Group on Nursing, *Toward Quality in Nursing: Needs and Goals*, Public Health Service Pub. #992 (Washington, D.C.: Government Printing Office, 1963), 22–23.

2   National Commission for the Study of Nursing and Nursing Education (Jerome Lysaught, Director), *An Abstract for Action* (New York: McGraw-Hill Book Company, 1970).

3   National Commission, *An Abstract for Action*, 155.

4   National Commission, *An Abstract for Action*, 89–90.

5   National Commission, *From Abstract into Action*, 89.

6   Roland H. Berg, "More than a Nurse, Less than a Doctor," *Look Magazine*, September 6, 1966, Freund Papers, Univ. of Penn.

7   Marianna Crane, "Olden Days of Nursing: Coronary Care Unit," *Nursing Stories (blog)*, July 21, 2020, nursingstories.org/2020/07/21/olden-days-of-nursing-coronary-care-unit/. Marianna Crane is also author of *Stories from the Tenth-Floor Clinic: A Nurse Practitioner Remembers* (Berkeley, CA: She Write Press, 2018).

8   Lawrence E. Meltzer, Rose Pinneo, and J. Roderic Kitchell. *Intensive Coronary Care: A Manual for Nurses*, 3rd ed. (Bowie, MD: Charles Press Publishers, 1977), i.

9   Paul J. Sanazaro, "The Research and Development Approach to Health Manpower," in

Joanna Buzek, ed., *Physician Support Personnel in the 70's: New Concepts* (Chicago: American Medical Association, 1971), 8.

10 American Medical Association, "Medicine and Nursing in the 1970s: A Position Statement," *JAMA* 213, no. 11 (September 14,1970):1881–83.

11 Barbara Bates, "Doctor and Nurse: Changing Roles and Relations," *New England Journal of Medicine* 283 (July 16, 1970): 129.

12 "AMA Urges New Major Role for Nurses," *American Medical News*, February 9, 1970; and "AMA Unveils Surprise Plan to Convert R.N. into Medic," *American Journal of Nursing Times* (1970): 691.

13 D. M. Storms and J. G. Fox, "The Public's View of Physician's Assistants and Nurse Practitioners," *Medical Care* 17 (1979):526–35; and Alfred Yankauer and Judith Sullivan, "The New Health Professionals: Three Examples," *Annual Review of Public Health* 3(1982): 249–76.

14 Natalie Holt, "'Confusion's Masterpiece': The Development of the Physician Assistant Profession," *Bulletin of the History of Medicine* 72, no. 2 (1998): 273–74.

15 Frankie Miller in discussion with the author and Booth, September 29, 1982, 1, Freund Papers, Univ. of Penn.

16 Frankie Miller, discussion, September 29, 1982, 1–2.

17 North Carolina Nurses Association, *Highlights in Nursing in North Carolina, 1935–1976* (Raleigh, NC: 1977), 17.

18 North Carolina Nurses Association, *Highlights in Nursing*, 17.

19 Frankie Miller, discussion, September 29, 1982, 2.

20 The Joint Practice Committee of North Carolina Medical Society and North Carolina Nurses Association published the following five task force reports in June 1978: Clinics Manned by Nurse Practitioners, Maternity and Family Planning, Occupational Health Services, Psychiatric–Mental Health, and Pediatric Nurse Practitioners. Another report, Emergency Nurse Clinician, was published in May 1978.

21 Betty Compton, discussion, December 16, 1982, 11.

22 Margaret Wilkman, discussion, September 29, 1982, 5–6.

23 Frankie Miller, discussion, September 29, 1982, 5–6.

24 Betty Compton, discussion, December 16, 1982, 13–14.

25 Some of the other North Carolina nurse practitioners attending one or both conventions included Hettie Garland, Connie Mullinix, Judy (Cheyunski) Roberts, and me.

26 Betty Compton, discussion, December 16, 1982, 14.

27 Fairman provides insightful background in her discussion of the conflict in ANA over its identity and purpose, and its struggles during the 1950s and 1960s, leading to its hesitancy in accepting nurse practitioners. Julie Fairman, *Making Room in the Clinic: Nurse Practitioners and the Evolution of Modern Health Care* (New Brunswick, NJ: Rutgers University Press, 2008), 114–33.

28 "Family Nurse and Pediatric Nurse Practitioners Consider Merging Their ANA Councils," *American Journal of Nursing* 75, no.11 (November 1975): 2076, accessed on July 24, 2020, journals.lww.com/ajnonline/Citation/1975/11000/ Family_Nurse_and_Pediatric_Nurse_Practitioners.6.aspx.

29 C. Glenn Pickard and Julia D. Watkins, eds., *Current Directions in Family Nurse Practitioner*

Curriculum: Proceedings of a National Conference of Representatives from Family Nurse Practitioner Programs, January 1976, Department of Health, Education, and Welfare Publication No. (HRA) 77-28 (Bethesda, MD: U.S. Department of Health, Education, and Welfare, 1977).

30 "History of NONPF," www.nonpf.org/page/1.

31 David Warren, discussion, September 28, 1982, 8.

32 North Carolina Board of Higher Education, North Carolina Medical Care Commission, and North Carolina State Board of Education, *Report of Survey of Nursing Education in North Carolina* (Raleigh, NC: 1964).

33 David Warren, discussion, September 28, 1982, 9.

34 Legislative Research Commission of the North Carolina General Assembly, *Report on the Shortages of Nurses and Other Medical Personnel in North Carolina, Report No. 10* (Raleigh, NC: 1967).

35 Legislative Research Commission of the North Carolina General Assembly, *Report of the Committee on the Physician Shortage in Rural North Carolina* (Raleigh, NC: 1969).

36 Legislative Research Commission of the North Carolina General Assembly, *New Categories of Health Manpower: Physician's Assistants* (Raleigh, NC: 1971).

37 Legislative Research Commission of the North Carolina General Assembly, *Report on the Lawful Role of the Nurse* (Raleigh, NC: 1973).

38 Legislative Research Commission of the North Carolina General Assembly, *Report on Physician's Assistants and Nurse Practitioners* (Raleigh, NC: 1977).

39 Audrey Booth and I interviewed the key nursing leaders at Duke—Thelma Ingles and Ruby Wilson, as well as Eugene Stead—about the nursing experiments conducted at Duke. Although not directly related to the development of the nurse practitioner movement in North Carolina at the time, their experiments were a significant attempt at enhancing nursing practice. Many nurse leaders in North Carolina were aware of these experiments, and they often arose in discussions of nurse practitioners. Appendix B includes a description of those experiments and the perspectives of Ingles, Wilson, Stead, and Estes (who succeeded Stead as chairman of family medicine). Natalie Holt also provides a description of the nursing experiments, the rejection of an innovative master's program by the National League for Nursing, and then the ultimate development of the PA Program at Duke, in Holt, "'Confusion's Masterpiece,'" 246–78, www.jstor.org/stable/44445024.\

40 Reginald Carter, "Biography of Ballenger, Martha D.," Physician Assistant History Society, 2012, pahx.org/ assistants/ballenger-martha-d/.

41 Harvey Estes, personal communication with the author and Booth, December 7, 1982, Freund Papers, Univ. of Penn.

42 California was the first state to enact enabling PA legislation in 1970.

43 David Warren, discussion, September 28, 1982, 26.

44 Glenn Pickard, discussion, August 26, 1982, 42.

45 Lucy H. Conant, Testimony to the Health Committee of the Legislative Research Commission, *New Categories of Health Manpower: Physician's Assistants* (North Carolina Legislature, May 1, 1970).

46 Glenn Pickard, Testimony to the Health Committee of the Legislative Research Commission, *New Categories of Health Manpower: Physician's Assistants* (North Carolina Legislature, May 1, 1970).

47 Glenn Pickard, discussion, August 26, 1982, 43–44.

48 Legislative Research Commission of the North Carolina General Assembly, *Report on the Lawful Role of the Nurse* (Raleigh, NC: 1973), 6.

49 Audrey Booth, personal communication to Freund, ~2016.

50 Legislative Research Commission of the North Carolina General Assembly, *Report on the Lawful Role of the Nurse* (Raleigh, NC: 1973), 31–32.

51 David Warren, discussion, September 28, 1982, 24.

52 The North Carolina Medical Society resolution presented to the commission in June 1972 is included in appendix F of the commission's report: Legislative Research Commission of the North Carolina General Assembly, *Report on the Lawful Role of the Nurse* (Raleigh, NC: 1973), 61.

53 Glenn Pickard, discussion, August 26, 1982, 42–43.

54 Glenn Pickard, discussion, August 26, 1982, 45.

55 Frankie Miller, discussion, September 29, 1982, 9–10.

56 Alok S. Patel, "Docs vs. NPs: How AMA Made Scope Creep Fight Uglier," *Medscape*, December 18, 2020.

57 David Warren, discussion, September 28, 1982, 20.

CHAPTER TEN

1 Alyssa LaFaro, "The Nursing Pioneer," March 15, 2017, *Endeavors* (blog), endeavors.unc.edu/the-nursing-pioneer/; G. I. Fitzgerald, *Pioneers*, 12 (unpublished), Freund Papers, Univ. of Penn.

2 Carolyn Williams, discussion, June 1, 1982, 27–28.

3 Glenn Wilson, discussion, September 27, 1982, 6.

4 Eugene Mayer in discussion with the author and Booth, December 2, 1982, 4–5, Freund Papers, Univ. of Penn.

5 Judy Watkins, discussion, November 9, 1982, 8.

6 James Bryan in discussion with the author, July 15, 2020, 23, Freund Papers, Univ. of Penn.

7 Glenn Wilson, discussion, September 27, 1982, 6. In this quote, Wilson is referencing the powerful figures in the medical school, the chairs of medicine and pediatrics.

8 Eugene Mayer, discussion, December 2, 1982, 6.

9 Glenn Pickard, discussion, August 26, 1982, 48.

10 Glenn Wilson, discussion, September 27, 1982, 4–5.

11 Cecil Sheps, discussion, June 1, 1982, 10.

12 Glenn Pickard, discussion, August 26, 1982, 17.

13 Glenn Wilson, discussion, September 27, 1982, 16.

14 Carolyn Williams, June 1, 1982, 12–13.

15 Glenn Pickard, discussion, August 26, 1982, 29.

CHAPTER ELEVEN

1 piedmonthealth.org/prospect-hill-location/, last accessed on June 4, 2021.

2 Brian Toomey (CEO of Piedmont Health), personal phone conversation with author, February 24, 2021.

3   Patricia Warren, personal conversation with the author at her home in Prospect Hill, April 7, 2021.

4   gchcinc.org, last accessed on August 28, 2020.

5   www.hotspringshealth-nc.org/about-us/history, last accessed on August 28, 2020.

6   www.ncahec.net, last accessed on August 28, 2020.

7   www.ncdhhs.gov/divisions/orh, last accessed on August 28, 2020.

8   Thelma Ingles and Ruby Wilson were the nursing faculty leading the way in these experiments. See Appendix A for more discussion on their clinical nursing experiments.

9   Linda A. McCauley, et al., "Doctor of Nursing Practice (DNP) Degree in the United States: Reflecting, Readjusting, and Getting Back on Track," *Nursing Outlook* 68 no. 4 (July 1, 2020): 494–503, doi.org/10.1016/j.outlook.2020.03.008.

10 Sharon K. Ostwald and Okwuoma Chi Abanobi, "Nurse Practitioners in a Crowded Marketplace: 1965–1985," *Journal of Community Health Nursing* 3, no. 3 (1986): 154, http://www.jstor.org/stable/3427523.

11 Cynthia M. Freund, "Research in Support of Nurse Practitioners," in eds. Diane O. McGivern and Mathy D. Mezey, *Nurses, Nurse Practitioners: Evolution to Advanced Practice* (Springer Publishing Incorporated, 1998), chapter 3, 59–87.

12 American Association of Nurse Practitioners, "NP Fact Sheet," AANP National Nurse Practitioner Database, 2020, www.aanp.org/about/all-about-nps/np-fact-sheet, accessed January 18, 2020.

13 David L. Auerbach, "Advanced Practice Provider Influx Will Reshape Primary Care," as reported by *Medscape Medical News*, June 20, 2018. Originally published by David L. Auerback, et al., *New England Journal of Medicine* 378 (2018): 2358–63.

14 Campaign for Action, AARP Foundation, AARP, and Robert Wood Foundation, "Issues: Campaign for Action Dashboard," updated January 4, 2021, campaignforaction.org/issue/improving-access-to-care/.

15 Lucille Sherman, "100 NC Lawmakers Signed onto a Health Care Bill. Then Donors Started Calling," *News&Observer*, April 4, 2021; www.newsobserver.com/news/politics-government/article250287935; Lucille Sherman, "Some Assembly Required: Lucille's Field Notes," Axios Raleigh, June 30, 2022, www.axios.com/newsletters/axios-raleigh-ee21d106-b8f8-4211-a131-3e479c70da3d; Gale Adcock, email message to author, July 2, 2022, Freund Papers, University of Pennsylvania. Patrick Ballantine, "Legislative Update 7/4/2022," NCNA Legislative Updates, ncnurses.org/advocacy/legislative/legislative-update-7-4-2211

APPENDIX A

1   All material related to the *North Carolina Nurse Practitioner Collection: The Freund–Booth Conversations with the Movement's Influential* are part of the Cynthia M. Freund Papers, The Bates Center for the Study of the History of Nursing, School of Nursing, University of Pennsylvania. Audrey Booth and I were the sole and principal interviewers.

2   Hereafter referred to as the *Conversations Collection*.

3   A few interviews were collected later between 2014 and 2018, during the initial phases of writing the book.

4 A few interviews were more formal, particularly when with those we had not worked with closely. But we knew the interviewee was involved in some important way in the early North Carolina NP movement, and thus felt it important to include them in the *Conversations Collection*. A prime example of this is the interview with former North Carolina Governor James E. Holshouser, Jr.

5 We did not start the tape recorder until all the salutary greetings and it's-good-to-see-you-again exchanges had been made. After preliminary information was shared and questions were answered, which included their consent to participate in the interview and our intent to use the material in writing a book about North Carolina's nurse practitioner movement, we started the tape recording. Their verbal agreement and actual participation in the interview were considered informed consent, quite acceptable in the early '80s. And whenever we were asked to stop the tape recorder so the interviewee could tell us something he or she did not want recorded, we did so without question or hesitation.

6 The unrecorded interview of Eugene Stead was unintentional. Due to some unknown technical glitch or user error, the tape recorder did not start and thus the interview was not recorded. Booth took notes at the meeting; I wrote a narrative summary after the meeting, capturing major points. These are included in the *Conversations Collection*.

7 In a few instances, because of a distant location of an interviewee, we sent a tape to the interviewee and asked them to record their recollections and perspectives, and then return the tape to us. Some chose to write in script their recollections and perspectives. This material is also included in the *Conversations Collection*.

APPENDIX B

1 See chapter 2.
2 Duke University School of Nursing, "History of Duke University's School of Nursing (Volume One: 1931 to 1971)," About Us, Our History, 2011, nursing.duke.edu/about-us/our-history.
3 Thelma Ingles, letter to Audrey J. Booth, September 9, 1982, 1, Freund Papers, Univ. of Penn.
4 Thelma Ingles, self-recorded tape provided to the author and Booth, August 1982, 2, Freund Papers, Univ. of Penn.
5 Thelma Ingles, tape, August 1982, 2.
6 Thelma Ingles, letter, September 9, 1982, 1.
7 Thelma Ingles, letter, September 9, 1982, 1.
8 Thelma Ingles, letter, September 9, 1982, 1.
9 Ruby Wilson in discussion with the author and Booth, December 10, 1983, 8, Freund Papers, Univ. of Penn.
10 Ruby Wilson, discussion, December 10, 1983, 7.
11 Ruby Wilson, discussion, December 10, 1983, 9.
12 Duke University School of Nursing, "History of Duke University's School of Nursing (Volume One: 1931 to 1971)," About Us, Our History, 2011, nursing.duke.edu/about-us/our-history, 23; and also corroborated by the taped discussion with Ruby Wilson on December 10, 1983, Freund Papers, Univ. of Penn.

13 Ruby Wilson, discussion, December 10, 1983, 10.

14 Ruby Wilson, discussion, December 10, 1983, 14.

15 Ruby Wilson, discussion, December 10, 1983, 14.

16 Harvey Estes, personal conversation, December 7, 1982, Freund Papers, Univ. of Penn.

17 Physician Assistant History Society, "Treadwell, Henry Lee 'Buddy,'" and "Johnson, Amos N.," Histories, Biographies, pahx.org/bio/.

INDEX

Page locators in italics indicate figures and tables

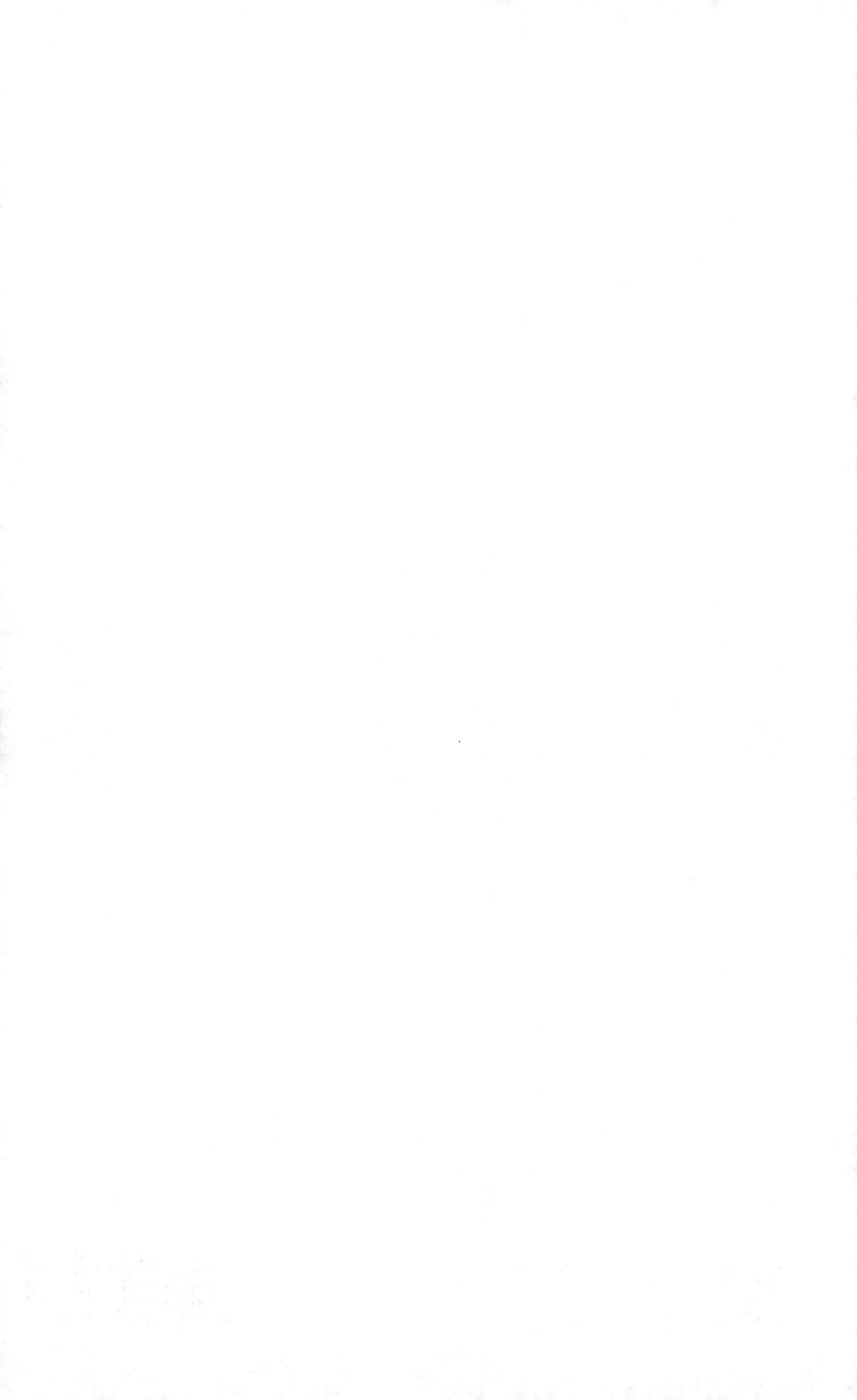

CPSIA information can be obtained
at www.ICGtesting.com
Printed in the USA
LVHW021915160822
726104LV00003B/267